Eat Smart Play Hard

Customized Food Plans for All Your Sports and Fitness Pursuits

LIZ APPLEGATE, Ph.D.

Author of *Power Foods*
University of California, Davis
Nutrition Department Faculty

RODALE

Notice

This book is intended as a reference volume only, not as a medical manual. The information given here is designed to help you make informed decisions about your health. It is not intended as a substitute for any treatment that may have been prescribed by your doctor. If you suspect that you have a medical problem, we urge you to seek competent medical help.

Cover and Interior Designer: Joanna Williams
Cover Photographers: Michael Keller/Corbis Stock Market, Mitch Mandel/Rodale Images, Scott Markewitz/FPG, Butch Martin/Image Bank, Steve Prezant/Corbis Stock Market, David Raymer/The Stock Market, Kurt Wilson/Rodale Images
Play Hard Pyramid graphic on page 4 designed by Glenn Hughes

Library of Congress Cataloging-in-Publication Data

    Applegate, Elizabeth Ann.
      Eat smart, play hard : customized food plans for all your sports and fitness
    pursuits / Liz Applegate.
      p.   cm.
      Includes index.
      ISBN 1–57954–344–8   paperback
      1. Nutrition.   2. Physical fitness.   3. Athletes—Nutrition.   I. Title.
    RA784 .A658 2001
    613.7—dc21   2001000205

Distributed to the book trade by St. Martin's Press

    6 8 10 9 7 5   paperback

Visit us on the Web at www.rodalesportsandfitness.com, or call us toll-free at (800) 848-4735.

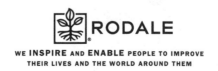

WE **INSPIRE** AND **ENABLE** PEOPLE TO IMPROVE
THEIR LIVES AND THE WORLD AROUND THEM

**To my mom, Marion, and my brothers and sisters:
Jim, Alice, Greg, Brien, Cathleen, Mike, Martin, and Chris**

Acknowledgments

My warmest thanks go to Alisa Bauman for her tireless editorial expertise and dedication. Without Alisa, I would be sunk! Also, many thanks to Marlia Braun for her professional assistance in the nutritional analysis of menus and recipes. And finally, to my husband, Mark, who never questions my endeavors.

Contents

Introduction

You play hard. Whether you spend all day on a golf course, hours in a bike saddle, 45 minutes at a local running trail, or a half-hour on a weight bench, you need to eat smart. Unfortunately, you have plenty of reasons to eat dumb.

Every day, people are misled by marketers and salesmen. Marketers have tried to convince fitness enthusiasts that they need juice from the stomachs of hornets to perform at peak levels. There have been media stories of athletes downing pickle juice to fend off heat cramps. And elite athletes have blamed common over-the-counter medicines for all sorts of performance pitfalls.

People also eat dumb because of outdated information. In the past decade alone, sports nutrition researchers have discovered hundreds of smarter eating strategies that can enhance your exercise program. Unfortunately, old habits die hard, and there are still plenty of coaches, journalists, and elite athletes spreading the old news that endurance athletes should subsist on bagels and pasta, that weight lifters should live on protein supplements, and that no athlete in his right mind should eat fat.

After helping hundreds of college and professional athletes, Fortune 500 company employees, university students, and regular folks, I realized that I needed to put all of this up-to-date information in one place so that even more people could benefit from it. My hope is that more people might eat smart.

In the pages of this book, I guarantee that you'll find more than a few surprises. Let me tell you about some of the major discoveries that have been made during the past decade in the field of fitness nutrition. A decade ago:

- Nutritionists began warning fitness enthusiasts to stay away from fatty foods such as nuts, avocados, olives, and salad dressings. For one, we thought they caused heart disease. But we also thought that fats had no place in a fitness diet. We couldn't have been more wrong. Researchers now know that special types of fats can prevent postexercise muscle soreness and the drop in immunity sometimes caused by too much endurance exercise. They may even prolong endurance. Plus, we also now know that certain fats can be kind to your heart.
- We believed that you could supply your body with all of the necessary vitamins, minerals, and other nutrients from food alone. Now we know that in some cases, that is simply not true. For example, food alone probably won't provide the nutrients you need to fend off joint pain after your workout; only a few specific supplements will do that. And food may not give you all the vitamin E you need to recover quickly enough for peak performance during your next exercise session.
- We boiled weight loss down to a simple equation: Burn more calories than you consume. That's still the case. But today we know more, especially about stubborn fat. Now, we know about specific foods that promote weight loss because they fill you up without filling you out. We also know about foods that speed your metabolism.

The list goes on. In each chapter of this book, you'll find out more about these advances and how you can use them to your advantage.

In part 1, New Fueling Basics, you'll find my exclusive Eat Smart Food Pyramid, a variation on the USDA's Food Guide Pyramid. My revised pyramid takes the government's pyramid and adapts it to the fit lifestyle. The USDA designed its food plan for couch potatoes, but people who play hard need more nutrients, fluids, and yes, fats. In this part, you'll also find the latest information on how to eat smart before, during, and after exercise. I also offer specific tips for pregnant and vegetarian fitness enthusiasts.

In part 2, Advances in Fitness Eating, I bring you the most up-to-date research on energy bars, energy gels, sports drinks, supplements, and performance foods. I tell you what works, what doesn't, and what falls somewhere in between.

In part 3, Eat to Reach Your Goals, you'll learn how to eat smart for 14 specific fitness pursuits. And that's the true beauty of the Eat Smart program. Other fitness books bring you a one-size-fits-all eating plan. But eating smart depends on your goals. A golfer simply doesn't have the same nutritional needs as a fitness walker or cyclist.

Within these chapters, you'll also get straight answers to frequently asked workout questions as well as news flashes about the latest fitness research and how to use it to your advantage. Finally, I include sample menus and recipes from my own food diary to help you prime your body to play as hard as you want.

So let's get started.

part one

New Fueling Basics

chapter one

The Play Hard Pyramid Plan

You are not the average person. You're the above-average person. You walk, swim, run, cycle, lift weights, play golf, or do some other type of physical exercise on a regular basis. You play hard, so you need more calories, more protein, and more nutrients than the average sedentary person. To know how much and what types of food *you* should eat, you need a different plan. That's why I designed the Play Hard Pyramid specifically for your fit lifestyle.

In 1992, the USDA unveiled its Food Guide Pyramid as a replacement for the outdated Four Basic Food Groups, which had been in place since the mid-1950s. The USDA based its pyramid design on the needs of average people, most of whom have no regular exercise program. The hope was that the pyramid would help put the government's dietary guidelines into common practice. Today, however, the Food Guide Pyramid is as outdated as the Four Food Groups. Numerous nutritional advances place the pyramid in desperate need of an overhaul, especially for the fitness-minded.

- The government placed all fats at the top of its pyramid in the "eat sparingly" section. Yet much research done since 1992 has found that not all fats are evil. In fact, many fats, such as the type found in chocolate, nuts, and cooking oils, are actually good for your

3

heart. Even more important, you need fats to fuel your active lifestyle. Research has found that the right types of fat will boost endurance and immunity and keep your joints well-lubricated. That's why I've split fats into two categories: healthful fats that you can eat three or more servings of a week, and unhealthful snack foods that you should eat sparingly.

- The government's pyramid lumps all carbohydrate into one big category at the base of the pyramid. Not all carbohydrate is created equal, however. Whole grains such as whole wheat bread, barley, quinoa, millet, and oatmeal provide nutrients that prevent sore muscles as well as heart disease. I've split the carbohydrate group in half to call attention to the whole grains. I've also bumped up

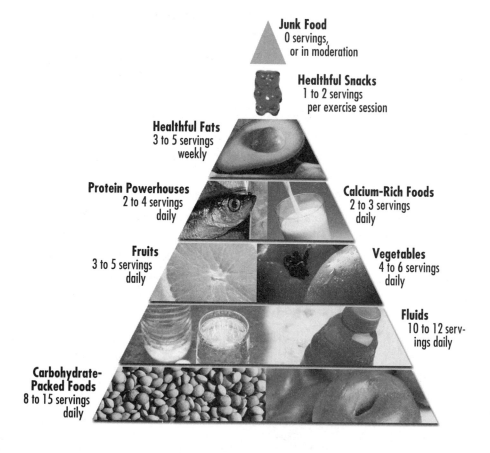

Junk Food
0 servings,
or in moderation

Healthful Snacks
1 to 2 servings
per exercise session

Healthful Fats
3 to 5 servings
weekly

Protein Powerhouses
2 to 4 servings
daily

Calcium-Rich Foods
2 to 3 servings
daily

Fruits
3 to 5 servings
daily

Vegetables
4 to 6 servings
daily

Fluids
10 to 12 servings daily

Carbohydrate-Packed Foods
8 to 15 servings
daily

your number of servings to 8 to 15, from the USDA's recommended 6 to 11 servings.

- The Food Guide Pyramid doesn't address the need for fluids. When you play hard, you sweat a lot, which is why I've put fluids close to the base of the Play Hard Pyramid.
- The USDA also doesn't include healthy snacks in its pyramid. Energy bars, gels, sports drinks, and performance foods such as Gummi Bears and fig bars deserve a spot on the Play Hard Pyramid.

In short, people who play hard need to eat smarter than the average couch potato. Keep the Play Hard Pyramid in mind when making your food choices each day. It should serve as a general guide, regardless of your age, gender, weight, or the type of exercise you're planning. You'll have to make some modifications based on these factors, and you'll find out how to do just that in the following chapters. Here's a closer look at the nine food groups that make up the Play Hard Pyramid.

The Nine Fitness Food Groups

The government's pyramid includes only six food groups. The Play Hard Pyramid bumps that number up to the following nine that are fine-tuned to meet your fitness needs.

Carbohydrate-Packed Foods

When you exercise, your muscles burn a type of carbohydrate called glycogen for fuel. To keep these important fuel levels optimal, you must eat a diet rich in grains, beans, potatoes, and other types of high-carbohydrate foods. Grains also contain important B vitamins such as thiamin, riboflavin, and niacin that your muscles need to convert the carbohydrate you eat into energy. Enriched refined grain products made from white flour, such as crackers, white rice, and pasta, do supply these B vitamins, but you should focus on whole grains such as whole wheat bread, quinoa, and brown rice, which also provide the fiber you need for a healthy heart and digestive tract. Despite popular belief, beans count as a high-carbohydrate food.

Amount needed: 8 to 15 daily servings. At least half of your daily

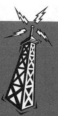

Nutrition News Flash

If you drink only bottled water, you're probably not getting enough fluoride. To strengthen tooth enamel and make it more resistant to tooth decay, your water should contain 1 milligram of fluoride per liter of water. Researchers at Case Western Reserve University in Cleveland and Ohio State University in Columbus sampled more than 50 brands of bottled water for fluoride content. They found that 90 percent of them had levels below the recommended range for dental health. On the other hand, when the researchers tested good old tap water, they found that it contained the ideal fluoride level.

servings should come from whole grains and at least five weekly servings should come from beans.

Fluids

The more you exercise, the more you sweat, and if you don't replace those lost fluids, you'll soon become dehydrated. Besides hurting your performance, chronic dehydration also increases your risk for kidney stones and bladder cancer. If you're watching your weight, go for water most of the time. During long workouts, however, you need a sports drink that contains carbohydrate and electrolytes.

Amount needed: 10 to 12 servings a day of water or other fluids such as fruit juice or sports drink.

Vegetables

Exercise makes you breathe hard; the harder you breathe, the more oxygen your lungs suck in. And while you need oxygen to sustain life, this gas tends to be unstable inside the body. Unstable oxygen molecules can oxidize, which may damage your muscle cells and set the stage for heart disease and cancer. Damaged muscle cells also bring on inflammation and soreness, which make your next workout feel harder than it should.

You can counteract oxidation by eating healthful amounts of antioxidants, substances found in dark, leafy greens; red peppers; tomatoes; winter squash; pumpkins; carrots; and other colorful produce. Fresh, frozen, or canned vegetables all supply a wealth of nutrients.

Amount needed: Four to six servings daily. Include two or more antioxidant-rich selections such as bok choy and spinach.

Fruits

Brightly colored fruits such as berries, kiwifruits, and oranges contain loads of antioxidants and other phytochemicals. Fruit juice counts, but you'll get more cholesterol-lowering fiber and other nutrients from whole fruits.

Amount needed: Three to five servings daily. At least half of them should be antioxidant powerhouses such as mango, pineapple, and cantaloupe.

Protein Powerhouses

Fit people need more protein (80 or more grams a day) than flabby people do. This macronutrient is especially important after your workouts, when your body repairs muscle damage and shuttles energy back to your muscles. So include soy, fish, eggs, and lean meat in your postworkout meals. Lean meat, especially beef, is loaded with zinc, a mineral that

---

Serving Sense

You might assume that you'll be stuffing yourself silly by eating 8 to 15 servings of high-carbohydrate foods. But a serving isn't nearly as large as most people think. Here are a few examples.

Group	Serving Size
Carbohydrate-Packed Foods	½ c cooked pasta, beans, couscous, or other grains (about the size of a computer mouse); one slice bread; ½ bagel; 1 oz cereal (see box for serving size)
Vegetables	1 c raw leafy greens (a little smaller than a softball); ½ c cooked or chopped raw vegetables
Fruits	1 medium piece of fruit (about the size of a tennis ball); ½–¾ c juice; ½ c chopped fruit
Calcium-Rich Foods	8 oz milk or soy milk; 1 c yogurt; 1½ oz cheese (about the size of three dice)
Protein Powerhouses	1 c soybeans; 2 soy burgers; 2–3 oz fish or lean meat (about the size of a deck of cards); 2 eggs
Healthful Fats	1 oz nuts (about 18 almonds); ⅛ avocado; 2 tsp oil

workout q&a

Q: • How bad is it to drink soda during exercise?

A: • It's pretty bad. Sodas have 12 to 15 percent carbohydrate by weight, which is much more than the suggested range of 5 to 9 percent. If you quaff a drink that has too much carbohydrate in it, you'll slow water absorption, which creates that sloshing feeling in your stomach.

most people need to get more of in their diets. And soy, fish, and other types of meat provide iron and other trace minerals such as copper and manganese that your body needs, especially during heavy training.

Amount needed: Two to four 2- to 3-ounce servings a day. Eat fish one or two times a week for its healthy omega-3 fats.

Calcium-Rich Foods

Consuming dairy products is the easiest way to ensure that you're getting plenty of bone-strengthening calcium. As a bonus, dairy products also offer a good dose of protein. If you don't eat dairy, select calcium-fortified soy products or other calcium-rich foods such as calcium-fortified orange juice or cereal. Aim for at least one soy product daily that supplies about 10 grams of protein.

Amount needed: Two to three servings daily.

Healthful Fats

The fat found in nuts, avocados, olives and olive oil, canola oil, and flaxseed and flaxseed oil is actually quite good for your heart. Additional research shows that these healthful fats may fight inflammation and muscle soreness and may even boost immunity.

Use healthful fats in place of heart-clogging saturated and trans fats such as margarine and butter. Snack on a handful of nuts instead of potato chips. Use avocado as a spread on bread instead of margarine or butter. Cook with olive or canola oil instead of margarine. And try flaxseed oil along with seasonings for an eat-smart salad dressing. Flaxseed oil also supplies a healthy dose of omega-3 fats, which are the same fats found in fish.

But be warned: All types of fat contain more calories per gram than either carbohydrate or protein do, so if you're watching your weight, you should watch your intake.

Amount needed: Three or more servings a week.

My Food Diary

I would never recommend something that I wouldn't do myself. That's why I took a day's worth of meals out of my food diary to show you what a typical day of fitness eating looks like for me.

Breakfast
1 cup cooked oatmeal topped with 8 ounces soy milk, one sliced banana, and 1 ounce walnuts

Morning Snack
8 ounces sports drink, one orange, and ½ whole wheat pita spread with 2 tablespoons hummus

Lunch
Two soy burger patties on a whole grain roll topped with tomato slices, lettuce, and onion; 1 cup fruit salad (berries, melon, kiwifruit); and 1 cup bean salad (black beans mixed with chopped peppers)

Afternoon Snack
1 cup plain yogurt mixed with ½ cup mixed dried fruit (apricots, raisins, papaya)

Dinner
Stir-fry containing 1 cup whole wheat soba (Asian-style) noodles, 3 ounces lean beef, and 1 cup chopped broccoli, yellow peppers, and snow peas; salad made of 1 cup spinach tossed with 2 teaspoons olive oil dressing, 1 ounce feta cheese, and 2 tablespoons toasted almonds

Evening Snack
2 cups popcorn and a cup of tea with 2 teaspoons honey

Calories: 2,500; Protein: 110 grams; Carbohydrate: 364 grams; Fat: 28% calories

Healthful Snacks

If you exercise for more than an hour at a time, you'll need to consume energy bars, gels, sports drinks, or other performance foods to fuel your fitness. Found in most grocery stores, health food stores, and sporting goods stores, products such as PowerBar, Gu, and Cliffshot contain easily digestible carbohydrate. They also make great pre- and postrun snacks. Most bars have 30 or more grams of carbohydrate; most gels contain about 25 grams. Foods such as Gummi Bears, fig bars, dried fruit, and honey also supply fast, digestible carbohydrate.

Amount needed: 30 to 60 grams per hour of exercise.

Junk Food

Chips, cake, soda, and doughnuts are not recommended foods. They offer too few nutrients and too many calories and are likely to contain either saturated or trans fats, two of your biggest artery cloggers. But let's face it, one of the reasons you exercise is to eat the foods you love. So munching on cookies or fatty snack foods now and then is not a huge deal as long as these foods don't become dietary staples.

Amount needed: One unhealthful snack or fewer per day.

Exercise Morning, Noon, or Night

The saying "Timing is everything" certainly holds true when it comes to hard play. I don't know about you, but once my schedule throws me a curveball, pushing my workout back 15 to 20 minutes, it becomes much more likely that I won't work out at all. When I do try to exercise at an unfamiliar time of day, my body doesn't always cooperate unless I change my nutritional habits to go along with the schedule change.

What and when you eat is closely connected to the time of day you exercise. People who work out first thing in the morning should eat differently than people who exercise on their lunch breaks. And those who play hard at noon need to follow a different nutritional program than those who sweat it out after work. Here are some factors to consider when planning your exercise program.

When to Work Out

The best time for you to work out depends on your specific exercise goal: general fitness, weight loss, conditioning for competition, or recreation. It's also important to recognize that your fitness schedule will be dictated to some degree by professional and family responsibilities as well as conditions that will fluctuate throughout the day, such as your environment, hormone levels, and sleep patterns. Here's how some of these factors influence your body's response to exercise.

Weight-loss wishes. Research suggests that the same workout may burn more calories in the morning than later in the day. Your body is relatively depleted of carbohydrate and energy after an overnight fast, so it burns more fat as fuel. But this doesn't mean you'll lose more weight. Exercise burns calories no matter what the time of day, and if you end the day eating fewer calories than you burned, you will lose weight.

Performance goals. If your exercise goals are centered around improving your strength, speed, or other performance issue, then a noon or afternoon workout may be best. Studies show that muscle strength is greatest at midday, and your ability to perform both aerobically (oxygen-using activities like jogging) and anaerobically (high-intensity activities like sprinting) peaks in the afternoon. Because your body temperature is a few degrees higher in the afternoon, however, the extra effort needed to handle the additional heat may minimize some performance benefits.

Heat worries. If overheating and sweating excessively makes working out no fun for you, opt for cooler times of the day. Morning and evening hours are best for outdoor exercises such as cycling, running, and soccer. A workout done in the heat may leave you dehydrated and weak, and your exercise session may not be as productive because of the heat stress.

Injury concerns. Many people believe that exercising in the morning leads to more injuries, but that isn't true. Despite the fact that many morning joggers stagger out the door half-asleep without even warming up, morning exercisers do not have greater injury rates than folks who work out in the afternoon or evening. Injury rates are more closely tied to how much exercise a person performs. And the relationship is a simple one: The longer you work out, the greater the likelihood of injury.

Sleep needs. The timing of your exercise can affect the quality of your sleep. Afternoon appears to be the best time to exercise if you want to promote a sound overnight slumber because your body's downward temperature cycle following a workout will coincide with bedtime, when your body temperature drops naturally. And a good night's sleep will make the next day's workout that much easier and enjoyable. Regular exercise also has been shown to decrease the amount of time needed to fall asleep.

Fresh-air priorities. Early morning, when traffic flow is light and the air is cleanest, is the best time for outdoor activities. Jog or walk around a track, on a trail among trees, or through open, green areas such as parks, especially if you live in an urban area. Breathing fresh air will help reduce oxidative damage to lung tissue caused by pollutants.

But the best time for you to exercise is when you can fit it in—morning, noon, or night. Exercising on the weekend is okay, too, although a daily workout is the better way to go. But no matter when you play hard, you need to eat smart to feel and perform your best. Follow the guidelines in the rest of this chapter, and you'll improve your workout in no time.

Morning Exercise

A peaceful walk at dawn. An early swim. A round of golf at sunrise. For morning types, there's nothing like the last hint of darkness and the first chirps of waking birds to accompany a workout. But not all fitness enthusiasts get moving early because they like it. For many, morning is the only time of day that's not already jam-packed with other tasks, or it's the only time that's not too hot to exercise outdoors.

Whatever your reasons, you must fuel up with the right foods and beverages. Eating before a workout—particularly food that supplies carbohydrate—performs two important functions. First, your muscles receive a supply of energy for powering your workout. Second, your entire body, especially your brain, gets the fuel and nutrients it needs for daily living.

Even so, eating too close to an exercise session may spoil your workout. Food or beverages in the digestive tract may cause discomfort, even cramping and nausea, as hard-working muscles divert your blood supply away from the intestinal tract.

And there lies the problem. It's hard enough getting out of bed early to burn a few calories. But getting out of bed a few hours early to eat, rest, and then exercise is asking too much for many people.

If you sleep until the last minute before you need to head out the door, you might not be able to fit in a preworkout meal without suffering some consequences. On the other hand, if you are a true early bird, you can chow down breakfast and then read the paper, fold some laundry, or even go back to sleep for an hour before your workout. Read the section that applies most to you, depending on your sleeping habits.

Morning Eating for Early Birds

If you are the type of person who can wake up to eat a couple of hours before your workout, try the following tips.

- Consume high-carbohydrate foods that are low in fat and have a moderate amount of protein. Carbohydrate-rich foods such as bread, cereal, pasta, fruit, and energy bars are digested relatively quickly; high-protein foods such as meat and fish and fatty foods such as full-fat dairy products take longer. An excellent choice for first thing in the morning is a whole grain bagel topped with tomato slices and reduced-fat cheese, or breakfast cereal and fruit with low-fat or fat-free milk or soy milk.
- Eat 400 to 800 calories in your preworkout meal. This amount should fuel your exercising body without making you feel sluggish or full. If you find that liquid sources of nourishment sit better in your stomach, wash down a piece of fruit or bread with a single can of a meal-replacement drink (about 300 calories).
- Drink at least 10 ounces of water or sports drink 2 hours before your morning exercise. This helps offset sweat losses during your workout and gives your kidneys time to rid your body of excess fluid.

Morning Eating for Late Sleepers

Despite everything that I preach, I can't get out of bed early enough to fuel up before my morning swim or run. And I know that there are plenty of other fitness enthusiasts out there in the same situation.

With only 10 minutes to chow down before revving up, the question arises: To eat or not to eat? That depends on your constitution as well as your fitness routine. For example, I can't stomach anything before swimming. Even a glass of juice can sometimes trigger heartburn or a stitch in my side, so I usually swim without eating. Are there consequences? Of course there are; if I got myself out of bed early enough to digest some calories, I would no doubt be able to swim longer and faster. On the other hand, I can usually gulp down half an energy gel just before my morning run.

Do some experimenting to see what you can stomach for different types of exercise. If you find that you can't stomach anything at all, just be sure to eat plenty for dinner the night before and for breakfast when you return home. Here are some small, easy-to-digest meals to try right before your workout.

- A meal-replacement drink; put one by your bedside and guzzle it after the alarm sounds
- A glass of sports drink
- A packct of cncrgy gcl
- A small fruit-flavored yogurt

Eating after Your Morning Workout

Many morning exercisers complain of ravenous hunger by midmorning and blame it on the exercise. Some of them even switch to a different exercise time to avoid that gnawing feeling. I tell them to blame what they ate (or didn't eat) for breakfast.

If your postworkout breakfast never satisfies you and you end up getting hungry later in the morning, you're not eating the right foods. A morning meal should supply at least one-quarter of your daily needs for calories, protein, fiber, essential fats, vitamins, and minerals. The problem is that cereal and juice are both high in carbohydrate, so they're quickly digested. And considering typical serving sizes, such a breakfast might be good for only a few hundred calories.

A smart postworkout breakfast supplies ample amounts of calories, protein, and fat. The protein and fat will slow digestion and keep you feeling full longer. As a result, you feel satisfied and ready to face your day. To achieve this goal, here are some suggestions.

- Sprinkle a handful of almonds or walnuts on your cereal for a dose of healthful fats and protein. Or spread peanut butter on a piece of whole grain toast and have it with your bowl of cereal.
- Try eggs in the morning. They're loaded with a wealth of nutrients such as protein, vitamin B_{12}, folic acid, vitamin K, and more. While you might think of eggs as a food to avoid, research shows no connection between egg consumption and blood cholesterol or risk of heart disease. In fact, egg eaters have been shown to have better overall nutrient intakes than those who avoid eggs.

Eating Smart for...
Morning Exercise

Here's a meal plan to keep you energized all day, despite an early wake-up call.

Preworkout Fueling
One energy gel pack
1 cup of coffee

Morning Workout

Breakfast
5-inch square flatbread spread with 2 tablespoons goat cheese sprinkled with 2 tablespoons dried cranberries and 1 tablespoon chopped almonds
One orange
4 ounces 1% milk or soy milk

Morning Snack
One cheese stick
Two whole wheat crackers

Lunch
1 cup minestrone soup
One slice whole wheat sourdough bread with 1 teaspoon trans-free margarine
10 baby carrots

Dinner
One beef kabob (3 ounces lean beef, mushrooms, onions, peppers)
¾ cup polenta
1½ cups greens with 1 tablespoon light ranch dressing

Calories: 1,705; Protein: 80 grams; Carbohydrate: 240 grams; Fat: 27% calories

- Avoid breakfast foods that traditionally accompany eggs. Sausage and bacon are loaded with artery-clogging saturated fat. Instead, try vegetarian sausage links made with heart-healthy soy protein. These are tasty and can be microwaved in seconds.
- Think outside the breakfast box. You don't have to stick with cereal and eggs. Try cottage cheese or yogurt topped with fresh fruits and

a handful of nuts, or cooked rice with raisins and soy nuts drizzled with honey. One of my favorite breakfasts is leftover pizza, usually a vegetarian variety with tomatoes and goat cheese. In fact, most leftovers make a great breakfast. Add a piece of fresh fruit for some added fiber and vitamins, and you're set for the morning.

Midday Exercise

I've always envied those lucky people who are either self-employed or who work for companies that encourage a fit lifestyle. I especially envy my colleagues at *Runner's World* magazine. Whenever I call one of them between 11:45 A.M. and 2:00 P.M., I'm met with voice mail and remember that they're all on a running break.

It's because of those editors that I decided to add this section. More and more companies are encouraging their employees to exercise during their lunch breaks. That's because these companies realize that fit employees are productive employees.

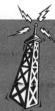

Nutrition News Flash

If you have trouble convincing your boss to give you a little extra time at lunch for your fitness program, give him this information: A study published in the *Journal of Occupational and Environmental Medicine* looked at the impact of the Citibank Health Management Program on changes in health risks among employees. Those who participated most in the program significantly lowered their health risks compared to those who participated least. If your boss wonders what this means to him, tell him that it means lower health insurance costs and fewer sick days.

Eating before Your Midday Workout

Many people who work out during their lunch breaks complain to me that hunger sometimes gets the better of them. That's because their breakfasts have been digested and processed and their blood sugar levels are starting to dip. Since the brain needs a steady supply of sugar, feelings of fatigue take over, making it difficult to muster the energy for a workout.

Rather than beefing up your breakfast, which may leave you feeling lethargic in the early morning, I recommend bringing a preworkout snack to munch on at work and following these eating tips.

Recipe Revver

Fudgy Wheat-Germ Brownies
Makes 12

On days when I exercise in the middle of the day, I find that a little chocolate treat keeps me focused at work. These brownies come with the goodness of wheat germ and walnuts as well as a good dose of protein, and are a good source of vitamins A and C, calcium, and iron.

  1 *package (6 ounces) semisweet chocolate chips*
  3 *tablespoons butter*
  ¾ *cup quick-cooking oats*
  ⅓ *cup toasted wheat germ (no sugar added)*
  ⅓ *cup nonfat dry milk*
  ½ *teaspoon baking powder*
  ½ *cup chopped walnuts*
  4 *egg whites*
  ½ *cup packed brown sugar*
  1 *teaspoon vanilla*

Preheat the oven to 350°F. Coat an 8" square baking dish with nonstick spray and set aside. In a microwaveable dish, melt the chocolate chips and butter at 85 percent power. Blend well and set aside.

In a small bowl, combine the oats, wheat germ, dry milk, baking powder, and walnuts.

In a large bowl, beat the egg whites with the brown sugar and vanilla until slightly thick. Stir in the chocolate mixture and then the oat mixture. Blend well, but do not overmix. Spread the batter into the prepared baking dish. Bake for 20 to 35 minutes, or until the edges are firm and the top is crisp. Cool completely before cutting, or refrigerate overnight before serving.

Per brownie: *221 calories, 6 g protein, 26 g carbohydrate, 12 g total fat, 5 g saturated fat, 9 mg cholesterol, 2 g dietary fiber, 57 mg sodium*

1. Avoid discomfort by eating 1 to 3 hours before your workout. This will allow sufficient time for your stomach to clear.
2. Eat 100 to 400 calories, depending on your body size and what you had for breakfast. If you ate a light breakfast—cereal and

juice, for example—you may want a bit more for your midmorning snack. But remember that you're snacking, not having a meal, which is usually 500 to 600 calories.

3. Consume high-carbohydrate, low-fat foods that can be easily digested. Eating a croissant 1 hour before exercising will make your gut feel like it's full of lead. Stay away from junk foods that are loaded with carbohydrate but offer little in the way of vitamins, minerals, or other vital nutrients.

Here are some snacks that are smart to munch before your next noontime workout. Try several of these suggestions to find the ones that work best for you, but whatever you do, don't let hunger foil your fitness plans, and be sure to wash down your food with plenty of fluids.

- ½ cup mixed dried fruit (apricots, raisins, papaya) with 6-ounce can of vegetable juice
- One slice of whole grain bread topped with 2 tablespoons fruit spread
- One breakfast bar
- 1 cup ready-to-eat breakfast cereal mixed with 3 tablespoons raisins
- One medium banana and three wheat crackers
- One package of instant oatmeal made with fat-free milk, soy milk, or water, and topped with honey and cinnamon
- One high-carbohydrate energy bar (no more than 4 grams of fat)

Eating after Your Midday Workout

The problem with exercising during your lunch hour is that you may not have time to eat lunch, which is an important meal. You need those calories to replenish spent glycogen stores in your muscles so that you can work out tomorrow during lunch without feeling pooped. Even without a lunchtime workout, you need those calories to fuel your brain for the rest of your workday.

To save time, pack your own lunch, especially if your company doesn't have a cafeteria. That doesn't mean lunch has to be boring or take all morning to make. Try these tips.

- Opt for convenience. If you shop smart for your lunch items, you won't have to spend much time assembling your lunch. Keep pack-

Eating Smart for...
Midday Exercise

Here's a 1-day meal plan fit for a noontime workout.

Breakfast
1½ cups oatmeal topped with 2 tablespoons raisins and 1 tablespoon chopped pecans
One orange
4 ounces 1% milk or soy milk

Morning Snack
½ pita spread with 1 tablespoon honey and ½ sliced banana

Noon Workout

Lunch
One bean-and-chicken burrito
2 tablespoons salsa
1 cup fruit salad

Afternoon Snack
¼ cup soy nuts and dried papaya
1 cup sports drink

Dinner
1½ cups Mexican casserole (corn tortillas, black beans, enchilada sauce, reduced-fat Cheddar cheese, and chile peppers)
2 cups spinach salad with 1 tablespoon oil and vinegar dressing

Calories: 1,990; Protein: 79 grams; Carbohydrate: 312 grams; Fat 23% calories

aged yogurts, raisins, nuts, baby carrots, cereal bars, and juice on hand to toss in your lunch bag.

• Throw in some fruit. To get a piece of fruit ready for your lunch bag, all you have to do is wash it.

• Think out of the box. Instead of the usual lunch meat sandwich, try spreading the bread with hummus and lining it with sliced tomatoes and cucumbers with sprouts. Or try peanut butter and jelly, an old childhood favorite. You can put pretty much anything between two slices of bread and have it taste fairly good.

- Make the most of leftovers. Any leftovers from dinner are fair game. And it's already in a container.
- Instead of one large lunch, consider all-afternoon snacking. Down a glass of sports drink or fruit juice as soon as you get back to your office and then nibble from there.

The Postworkout Slump

Some people who exercise during their lunch breaks complain to me that they feel like taking a nap soon after their workouts. It's possible that these same people would experience a midafternoon slump even if they didn't work out during lunch. In other words, the slump may not be caused by exercise. Regardless of what causes it, here are some ways to stay energized.

1. Check your hydration level. A hard workout on a hot day can leave you dehydrated, which can lower your mental performance for the rest of the afternoon. Be sure to drink plenty of fluids throughout the morning before your exercise session, and have at least two generous glasses of water or sports drink afterward.

2. Have some protein. A high-carbohydrate meal—pasta, bread, and fruit, for example—can alter levels of the brain neurotransmitter serotonin, causing feelings of calmness and even drowsiness. But adding protein such as tofu or seafood to your lunchtime pasta can provide the right mix of nutrients in the blood, including amino acids, which alter brain neurotransmitter levels to boost alertness.

3. If you're ravenous just after your workout, you may overeat, which pulls blood to your stomach and away from your brain. Instead of gulping down everything in your lunch bag all at once, try snacking throughout the afternoon.

4. Take a break. A walk around the building, some stretches in the hallway, or a casual chat with a coworker may be all you need to get yourself going again.

Evening Exercise

After a stressful day at the office, there's nothing like a brisk walk or bike ride to burn up excess adrenaline. The problem is that sometimes you don't feel like heading out the door for that walk. You may be hungry or just plain beat. There's also the danger that when you come back from exercising, you'll be so famished that you eat everything you can find as you make dinner, which might not be on the table until 8:00 P.M. And the last thing you want to do is go to bed with a full stomach. Fortunately, these challenges can be met easily by eating smart before and after your evening exercise.

Eating before Your Evening Workout

To make sure you have enough fuel for your workout and enough calories left after exercise to prevent overeating, heed the following suggestions.

1. Never skip breakfast. Try cereal topped with a few walnuts along with milk and an orange, for example. Or blend up a smoothie made with yogurt, fruit, juice, and ice and take it with you on your commute. Your goal is take in at least 500 calories in the morning.
2. Make lunch your main meal of the day. Consume high-quality protein, such as fish, chicken, tofu, lean beef, or cooked beans with a grain (such as a bean burrito) along with fresh fruit and vegetables.
3. Have a midafternoon snack of fruit, pretzels, or an energy bar along with some water to ready yourself for your workout.

Eating after Your Evening Workout

Always eat after your workout, no matter how late it is. Your body needs nutrients such as carbohydrates and protein to recover. Many people worry about eating too close to bedtime because they fear that the calories will go straight to their fat cells while they sleep, but this isn't true. After exercise, your muscles need to restock glycogen, so they will absorb calories even while you're asleep, storing them to be burned during your next workout. Those calories will turn to fat only if you overeat, which you can avoid with the help of the following tips.

1. As soon as you walk in the door after your workout, guzzle some fluid, such as mineral water with a squeeze of lime. As you prepare your food, keep drinking. This will replace sweat losses and help you fill up.

2. Keep your evening meal light. Try a stir-fry with tofu, seafood, or lean meat over wheat noodles or rice along with fresh fruit. A sandwich (tuna with sprouts on whole grain bread) along with a piece of fruit would be an excellent post-workout meal before bedtime. Vegetable soup and crackers, or a frozen dinner with 500 calories or less would also be good choices. The key is to have foods on hand that you can easily prepare in small portions. This way, you can avoid what I call ravenous rage: eating anything in sight. You'll sleep better, too.

A Word on Frozen Dinners

If, at the end of the day, after your workout, you have no time or energy to cook, try a frozen entrée. You may have thought frozen dinners were bad news, but with a little sprucing up, you can turn a frozen meal into a nutrient-packed dining experience in a matter of minutes.

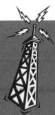

Nutrition News Flash

"Don't exercise too close to bedtime, or you'll have trouble falling asleep." This warning seems to make sense because exercise speeds up your heart rate, makes you sweat, and generally makes you feel more alert. Not everything that seems like common sense is actually true, however.

"Yes, exercising close to bedtime still might impair sleep for some less fit individuals, but not for everyone," says Shawn D. Youngstedt, Ph.D., a researcher at the University of California, San Diego, who put this theory to the test. He asked 16 people to cycle vigorously for 3 hours, finishing just a half-hour before hitting the sack. The cyclists fell asleep just as quickly as on nights when they watched television or read before bedtime. "We tested highly trained athletes who have a quicker physiological recovery following exercise than less fit people do," says Dr. Youngstedt.

So the bottom line is that unless you're just starting an exercise program, working out in the evening probably won't impair your sleep.

Eating Smart for...
Evening Exercise

Use this menu as a guide, and you'll never be too hungry to work out or too full to fall asleep.

Breakfast
> Smoothie made with 1 cup frozen mixed berries, ½ banana, ¾ cup low-fat vanilla
> yogurt, 4 ounces cranberry juice, and ice

Morning Snack
> One whole wheat bagel spread with 2 tablespoons almond butter

Early-Afternoon Lunch
> "Works" burrito (½ cup black beans, ½ cup rice, chopped tomatoes, romaine lettuce,
> 2 tablespoons grated Cheddar cheese, ⅛ avocado, 1 large flour tortilla) served with
> 1 cup apple-raisin-walnut salad and iced tea

Midday Snack
> 1 ounce pretzels
> 12 ounces water

After-Work Workout

Late Dinner
> Frozen entrée: chicken primavera (chicken and veggies over rice)
> Chopped radishes and broccoli dipped in 2 tablespoons light ranch dressing
> One chocolate biscotto cookie

Calories: 1,920; Protein: 75 grams; Carbohydrate: 280 grams; Fat: 29% calories

1. Check the **calorie count** on your frozen entrée. Aim for 300 to 500 calories. Considering that adults need about 2,000 calories daily, the 500-calorie limit will help you avoid overeating, especially if you add extras such as before-dinner snacks or salads.

2. Eye the total fat and saturated **fat content** of your selection. Aim for no more than 15 grams of total fat and 5 grams of saturated fat per frozen entrée or meal. If you include a salad or other low-fat add-ons like steamed veggies, your meal will take on an even healthier fat profile.

3. Setting a **sodium** limit can be tricky because most processed foods, including frozen entrées, come with plenty of added sodium. Your daily limit is 2,400 milligrams, and most frozen entrées have 300 to 900 milligrams of sodium. I wouldn't worry about the sodium content too much if your blood pressure is normal, however.

4. The **sugar content** of most frozen meals isn't a health issue, although the dessert that is included has added sugar. Too much sugar detracts from your intake of other nutrients, so you're better off adding your own dessert (see tips below).

5. Check the **fiber figure** for your entrée. Vegetarian lasagna or a vegetable stir-fry provides 3 to 6 grams of fiber. Your daily goal is a minimum of 25 grams, so select a frozen entrée with about 5 grams of fiber, or 20 percent of the Daily Value listed on the entrée's packaging. This is especially important if your fruit and vegetable intake is skimpy.

To round out your healthy heat-up meal without adding much in the way of preparation time, here are some easy-to-follow tips.

- Keep bagged salad mix on hand (specifically a spring mix type with dark, leafy lettuce) to make a quick side salad to go with your entrée.
- While heating your meal in the microwave, munch on precut fresh vegetables dipped in reduced-fat salad dressing or hummus.
- Along with your entrée, microwave a vegetable such as cauliflower, green beans, broccoli, or asparagus in a covered dish for extra fiber, vitamins, and minerals.
- Finish your meal with a healthy dessert of fresh berries topped with a touch of light whipped cream or yogurt. Frozen fruit sweetened with a drizzle of honey is also easily prepared and loaded with vitamins. Or try an apple microwaved in a covered dish served with raisins and cinnamon.

The Weekend Warrior

There are those of you who *want* to exercise regularly during the week. You really do. But the workouts just never seem to happen. The

Eating Smart for...
A Wild Weekend

Follow this menu on "warrior day" to boost your exercise recovery.

Breakfast
Three 6-inch buckwheat pancakes topped with ¾ cup fresh blueberries and 2 tablespoons
    maple syrup
8 ounces 1% milk

Morning Workout

Lunch (take along to park)
Turkey wrap (3 ounces roasted turkey, ¼ cup shredded carrots, 1 ounce provolone
    cheese, spinach leaves, mustard, 2 teaspoons fat-free mayonnaise, 1 large
    tortilla)
10 radishes or baby carrots dipped in 1 tablespoon light ranch dressing
Two oatmeal cookies

Midday Snack
One energy bar
8 ounces sports drink

Afternoon Workout
One energy gel pack
8 ounces sports drink

Dinner
4 ounces grilled lean beef
Eight spears asparagus
1 cup wild rice
Two slices whole wheat sourdough bread
1 ounce chocolate candies

Calories: 2,480; Protein: 112 grams; Carbohydrate: 350 grams; Fat: 26% calories

alarm goes off early in the morning for that before-work jog, but you turn
it off and go back to sleep. You plan to hit the gym during your lunch
break, but your 11 o'clock meeting runs late. After work, you simply
don't feel like it, and opt to relax with a beer instead of a bike ride.

Maybe tomorrow, you tell yourself. Eventually, Friday rolls around and "maybe tomorrow" is a must. When Saturday dawns, out come the inline skates, hiking boots, or rock-climbing shoes.

You usually feel great on Saturday. After being cooped up in an office all week, you're happy to be outside with the wind in your hair and the sunshine on your skin. On Sunday, you feel a little sore, but you feel like you might as well play some more before sitting on your butt at work tomorrow.

Then you wake up on Monday with the weekend warrior's hangover. Headache. Lethargy. Soreness. Not from drinking, mind you (although sometimes that's the case as well), but from pure, simple exertion.

When your weekend workouts go beyond your body's fitness level, it's no wonder that you struggle through Sunday's efforts and feel even more wrung out at work the next day. A smart eating plan will go a long way toward preventing the Monday-morning hangover. But the most important thing you can do is fit in some fitness during the workweek. If you don't, your body detrains, losing some of the fitness benefits gained over the weekend. It's as if you were starting over each weekend.

Instead of cramming a week's worth of workouts into just 2 days— which strains your muscles and joints and contributes to fatigue and muscle soreness—try squeezing in one or two sessions of aerobic exercise on the weekdays. Aim for 30 minutes per session at about 75 percent of your maximum effort. You want a workout that is vigorous but not completely exhausting. A spin on a stationary bike, a session on the stair-stepper, or a half-hour run will help you build a fitness base that will make your weekend workouts not only more doable but also more enjoyable.

Eating before Your Weekend Workout

Your weekend blowout sessions bleed your muscles of their stored carbohydrate energy (glycogen), which leads to that drained feeling on Sunday and Monday. You're sweating out fluids, too, which adds to fatigue if you don't replenish them. To combat these and other bodily enemies of the weekend warrior, eat smart during the week. Prepare yourself for your weekends by stocking your body with carbohydrates and fluids.

1. Eat an abundance of high-carbohydrate foods during your work-week, including cooked whole grains (brown rice, couscous), fruits, and vegetables.
2. Avoid skipping meals on Friday, which will drain your glycogen stores.
3. Hydrate yourself well on Thursday and Friday by drinking lots of water. Keep a bottle at your desk and sip from it frequently.
4. Go easy on the caffeine. Coffee, tea, and cola all dehydrate you to some degree, so keep tabs on how much of these you drink.

During your workouts, make sure to drink plenty of water. For workouts lasting more than 90 minutes, use a sports drink. These beverages contain carbohydrate to help stave off fatigue, and small amounts of electrolytes like sodium that encourage you to drink more fluid, which keeps your performance high and your threat of dehydration low.

Eating after Your Weekend Workout

After each weekend workout, prime yourself for the coming week by following these tips to help speed your recovery.

1. Drink plenty of fluids immediately after your workout to offset sweat losses. Aim for 16 ounces of water or sports drink for every 30 to 45 minutes you exercised.
2. Hit the carbohydrate soon after exercise to replenish spent glycogen stores. Plan on eating about 1 gram of carbohydrate for every pound of body weight within 30 minutes of finishing your workout.
3. Add some protein into your postworkout meal to further boost your glycogen rebuilding. A tuna sandwich with a piece of fresh fruit, or a fruit smoothie made with yogurt, soy milk, or protein powder both make great recovery meals.

With these exercising and eating strategies, your weekend play will be far more enjoyable, and when Monday comes, you'll feel great.

chapter three

Eat Smart
before Exercise

I have lost count of the number of workouts that have been cut short by new fitness buddies who don't eat smart. The scenario typically goes something like this: My food-deprived buddy and I go for a run. Only a mile or two out, my friend starts to complain that she isn't feeling well. "I guess today's not going to be a good run. I should probably turn back."

"Did you eat anything before the run?" I ask.

"I ate plenty. I had a bagel for breakfast."

"That's it?"

"What do you mean, 'That's it?' I usually don't eat breakfast at all."

At that point, I know that my would-be running mate has a lot to learn before she will be able to keep up.

There are plenty of runners, walkers, cyclists, swimmers, and other fitness enthusiasts out there making the same mistake of dieting and upping mileage at the same time. I'm here to tell you that unless you eat right before exercising, you'll never have a good day. Your workouts will always be cut short with complaints of light-headedness, fatigue, and nausea.

Why Eating Is So Important

Like many people, you may think that eating before exercise is self-defeating. After all, if you work out to lose weight, why would you want to

workout q&a

Q: Whenever I eat before working out, I feel sick during the workout. I even throw up sometimes. What do you suggest?

A: If you feel your food coming back up, you probably made one of three errors—or all three. You ate too soon before exercising, you ate too much food, or you ate food that had too much fat or protein, both of which slow digestion.

Food or beverages in the digestive tract may cause discomfort or even cramping and nausea during exercise, as your hard-working muscles divert blood supply away from the intestinal tract, slowing digestion. Depending on what you eat—high-carbohydrate versus high-protein or high-fat foods—the digestion process takes 2 hours or more. Most carbohydrate-rich foods, such as bread, cereal, pasta, fruit, and energy bars, are processed quickly. High-protein foods such as meat and fish take a bit longer. Fatty foods, including rich desserts, full-fat dairy products, and fried foods, take hours.

Start with a sports drink, which is designed to move through your gut quickly. Try to drink an entire 16-ounce bottle 1 to 2 hours before you exercise. Once you get used to that, move on to semi-solid foods such as nonfat fruit-flavored yogurt, jelly, honey, and applesauce.

counteract all of those burned calories by filling your body with food? There are plenty of reasons.

1. You'll actually burn *more* calories by eating before you run, swim, walk, or lift weights. When you don't eat before your workout, many of the reasons for exercising—conditioning, fitness, building muscle mass and strength, losing weight—go out the window. That's because your body turns to muscle protein for fuel when it doesn't have enough carbohydrate to burn. If you start your workout well-fueled, your body will burn a combination of the carbohydrate stored in your muscles *and* fat stored in your fat cells.

2. You'll have the motivation to get out the door. If you work out during your lunch break or after work, you're probably all too fa-

miliar with the excuses "I'm too hungry" and "I'm too tired."

3. You'll have the endurance to lengthen your workout. How many times have you stopped exercising because you felt dizzy, shaky, or just plain pooped? That's because you didn't have enough fuel to go the distance.

4. You'll perform better. Stocking up on food delays that burning feeling in your muscles, which will help you run, cycle, walk, or swim faster and for longer periods of time. Test subjects who ate before exercising also reported feeling better and rated their efforts as less rigorous than those who had fasted beforehand.

5. Your body needs fuel to keep your heart pumping and your brain buzzing even when you're not pounding the pavement. Have you ever felt light-headed when you haven't eaten for several hours? That's a sign that your brain is suffering from less-than-ideal fueling conditions. The bottom line is that you need to eat every 3 to 5 hours to maintain basic body functions.

Eating smart before a workout—particularly food that supplies loads of carbohydrate—provides a whole host of benefits. Your muscles receive an infusion

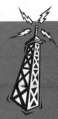

Nutrition News Flash

If you want to lose weight, increase the intensity of your workouts. I don't know how many times I've cringed as I overheard some so-called fitness expert telling people to exercise long and slow for the best fat-burning. It's true that you burn less fat and more carbohydrate during an intense workout than during moderate exercise. But the fact is that intense exercise usually burns more total calories, especially after the workout.

Consider the results of a study published in *The Journal of Sports Medicine and Physical Fitness*. Researchers in Seoul, Korea, asked men to exercise at varying intensities and durations, then measured their body temperatures and oxygen consumption for 2 hours following the workout. Short-duration exercise such as soccer or tennis burned more fat after the activity ended than longer, slower efforts did.

But crank up the intensity all the time only if you enjoy it. After all, the best form of exercise is the one that you will do most often, not the one that you dread.

Recipe Revver

Kiwi Salsa
Serves 6

This salsa not only tastes great on everything from fajitas and fish to baked potatoes but also is loaded with nutrients that can keep you healthy and exercising longer.

2   medium kiwifruits, peeled and diced
1   small red onion, chopped
1   red bell pepper, seeded and chopped
1   clove garlic, crushed
⅓   cup chopped fresh cilantro
2   tablespoons pineapple or lemon juice
¼   teaspoon red pepper flakes

In a medium bowl, combine the kiwis, onion, bell pepper, garlic, cilantro, pineapple or lemon juice, and red pepper flakes. Be sure to distribute the red pepper flakes evenly throughout the mixture. Chill before serving.

Per serving: 30 calories, 1 g protein, 7 g carbohydrate, 0 g total fat, 0 g saturated fat, 0 mg cholesterol, 2 g dietary fiber, 0 mg sodium

of energy to help maximize the results of your workout, and your entire body (especially your brain) gets the fuel and nutrients it needs for daily living.

What, When, and How Much

Here's a look at specific eating guidelines for preworkout fueling.

1. Eat 2 to 4 hours before a workout. This may mean planning your meals at different times to accommodate your workout schedule. For example, you may eat lunch at 2:00 P.M. so you can work out at 6:00 P.M.

2. Eat 400 to 800 calories at your pre-exercise meal. This amount should fuel your workout without making you feel sluggish or full.

3. Choose high-carbohydrate foods that are low in fat and have a moderate amount of protein. A whole grain bagel topped with tomato

slices and low-fat cheese, or breakfast cereal and fruit with 2% milk or soy milk, are both excellent choices.

4. Drink at least 10 ounces of water or sports drink 2 hours before you exercise. This helps offset sweat loss during your workout. The 2 hours gives your kidneys time to rid your body of any excess fluid.

12 Snacks to Get You Energized

Try one of the following great preworkout snacks 2 hours before your next run, bike ride, or swim.

- 6 ounces vegetable juice and ½ cup dried apricots
- A high-carbohydrate energy bar (look for one with 40 grams of carbohydrate and fewer than 3 grams of fat)
- One piece whole grain pita topped with 3 tablespoons fruit spread
- One glass sports drink and 1 cup ready-to-eat, whole grain breakfast cereal mixed with 1 tablespoon raisins
- One package instant oatmeal made with 4 ounces vanilla soy milk or fat-free milk with a dash of cinnamon and sugar

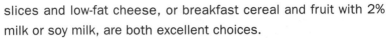

My Food Diary

When I agreed to actually write what I eat for the entire world to see, I honestly didn't realize how embarrassing it would be. After all, no one is perfect. Even though I strive to eat the foods that I recommend to others, I slip up from time to time. And my before-exercise eating is no exception. I simply have not found a way to eat much before my morning runs and swims. But later in the day, for my long bike ride, I have no trouble fueling. Here's what works for me.

Before running or swimming. Most foods don't sit well in my stomach during a morning run or swim (and because I go swimming first thing in the morning, I don't have much time to eat), so I usually drink a nonfat latte and nibble on some bread. Because I keep my runs under 45 minutes, I can survive. If I wanted to run longer, I'd have to add calories, perhaps from an energy gel.

Before cycling. I usually consume 800 to 1,000 calories before starting my 4-hour bike rides. This meal often consists of a whole wheat bagel with peanut butter, a banana, and an orange. Sometimes, I also eat an energy bar.

- One toasted plain bagel with 2 teaspoons jam, a banana, ½ cup cooked rice sprinkled with cinnamon, and 8 ounces sports drink
- A 1½-ounce box of raisins
- Two mini bagels spread with low-fat cream cheese mixed with 2 tablespoons dried cherries
- 6 ounces applesauce poured over three 3-inch squares of cornbread and topped with 2 tablespoons raisins
- One cup sliced banana in vanilla yogurt
- 10 chocolate animal crackers and a glass of cranberry juice
- One cup cooked pasta tossed with ½ cup dried cranberries and 2 tablespoons honey

Fueling for a Morning Workout

If you work out first thing in the morning, you may have a tougher time fueling simply because it's hard to jump out of bed, slam down breakfast, and then head straight out the door without avoiding tummy trouble. But you should never exercise on a completely empty stomach. Fueling for a morning workout requires two plans: a nighttime eating plan and a morning eating plan. Let's first look at what you should eat the night before your morning workout.

Dinner. I usually tell people to eat a huge breakfast, a somewhat lighter lunch, and a very light dinner, but morning exercisers should flip this upside down. You should fuel up with a large high-carbohydrate dinner to fully stock the fuel tanks in your muscles for the next morning's exercise. For example, try pasta with tomato sauce, a salad, and some bread, or a veggie stir-fry with rice.

Breakfast. Since you're eating so close to the time that you will exercise, you don't want to eat too much. Try to get in at least 100 calories. You'll have an easier time with stomach jostling if you make your calories liquid. Try a sports drink, a meal-in-a-can (such as Carnation Instant Breakfast), a glass of orange juice, or a packet of energy gel.

You're also better off choosing a type of morning exercise that doesn't jostle your belly. For example, cycling and walking are easier on the stomach than swimming and running. That doesn't mean you can't swim or run, it just means you'll have to experiment with your fueling plan.

Eat Smart
during Exercise

f you're like the majority of fitness enthusiasts, you work out moderately for less than an hour at a time. You've probably never eaten during exercise, and you don't need to start now.

But if somewhere in the back of your mind you think that you might want to challenge yourself by training for a century bike ride, a 2-mile swim, an all-day hike, or a 13-plus-mile run, then eventually you must learn how to eat and exercise simultaneously. And if you play sports that require short bursts of energy, such as soccer or racquetball, eating during exercise, while not required, can boost your performance.

Even if you're content to exercise moderately for less than an hour a day for the rest of your life (a perfectly healthy thing to do), you still should drink plenty of fluids during exercise, especially on hot days. Here's why.

1. You lose fluid through sweat and breath. As soon as you start to dehydrate, your body responds by working harder. Your heart rate increases, your muscles become starved for oxygen, and your performance suffers.
2. Your body drains stored carbohydrate from your muscles as you exercise. After about 90 minutes, your body runs out of this fuel and you start to crash. As your muscles pull sugar out of your blood-

35

stream, your liver attempts to replace it but soon runs out of glycogen itself. Once your blood sugar falls, you bonk, (an affectionate term for the light-headed, nauseated, and weak feelings that follow).

3. If you rely only on water for ultra-endurance events, you're not replacing the sodium that you lose in your sweat. For most people who exercise for an hour or less, this isn't a problem. But for exercise that is longer in duration, such as a marathon, you can run dangerously low on sodium. Too little sodium sets off a dangerous blood-electrolyte imbalance that mimics the symptoms of dehydration: headache, dizziness, and nausea. Left untreated, this can be life-threatening. Sports drinks, energy bars, energy gels, and fitness water, along with food, all contain enough sodium to prevent this problem.

The Three Vital Elements

Depending on the weather and the duration and intensity of your workout, you may need to supplement your consumption of one, two, or all three of these vital elements: fluids, carbohydrate, and electrolytes. Whether you stick with water or move on to sports drinks and energy bars to support your hard play takes careful consideration. To help you eat smart, here's a closer look at how each element functions in the body.

Fluids

The moment you start exercising, your body begins losing water through sweat, and this fluid loss quickly compromises performance. Your exercising muscles generate heat that your body must get rid of—or overheat. But as you sweat in an effort to stay cool, your cardiovascular system gets stressed because of the dropping water levels in your body.

Research has shown that every liter of sweat lost translates to an eight-beats-per-minute increase in heart rate. You can lose a liter of fluid in as little as 30 minutes, depending on the heat, humidity, and your sweat rate. If you don't replace that lost fluid, you put undue stress on your heart and internal cooling system. As a result, your core body temperature climbs, your performance plummets, and you risk serious heat illness. And even slight dehydration will hinder your performance.

For longer workouts, especially if you sweat heavily, try to match your fluid loss with your intake. This means drinking 5 to 12 ounces of fluid every 15 minutes of exercise. That sounds like a lot, and most people don't manage it. (Surveys show that most people consume a measly 8 ounces an hour, which amounts to just 30 percent of sweat loss.) But with practice, you can train yourself to do it. If you switch from water to either sports drink or fitness water (see "Fitness Water" on page 100), you'll automatically drink more. Studies show that people consistently consume more of a flavored beverage than they do of water. If you exercise for an hour or less, try fitness water, which contains plenty of flavor but very few calories per serving.

Carbohydrate

Studies show that consuming some form of carbohydrate as little as a half-hour into your workout can help you exercise longer and more intensely, especially if your session will last 90 minutes or longer. That's because carbohydrate keeps your blood sugar levels steady, which in turn helps your muscles access more fuel. As an added benefit, regular carbohydrate consumption also keeps your immunity high. (Some studies show that immunity plummets with long, intense exercise such as marathoning and century riding unless you eat carbohydrates during the exercise.)

What exactly is a carbohydrate? It's sugar, pure and simple. While you may be thinking of the white sugar in the bowl on your kitchen table, carbohydrate sugars come in many forms with complicated names such as glucose, sucrose, maltodextrin, and fructose. Carbohydrate is found in everything from bagels to pasta to sports drinks.

To be smart, consume 30 to 60 grams of carbohydrate for every hour of exercise. That comes to 120 to 240 calories per hour. The key is to keep a steady supply of carbohydrate entering your bloodstream. If you wait for an hour before you start to eat, it's too late. Your goal is to consume 60 to 120 calories every half-hour, with the specific amount varying according to body size and exercise intensity.

workout q&a

Q: I never eat while I run because it always makes me feel sick. Any suggestions?

A: You'll need to experiment, since no single food works for everyone. Try liquids first. Sports drink travels through your stomach faster than solid food does, so that's your best choice during exercise. If one sports drink doesn't work for you, try another. Different drinks contain different amounts of sugar, and some have additives or flavoring that could be making you feel sick. Take a walking break while you drink to eliminate sloshing, and take smaller, more frequent sips.

Exactly what you eat during your workout is a matter of personal preference, but it should be high in carbohydrate and low in fat, protein, and fiber. Here are some popular options.

Sports drinks. Hundreds of companies make sports drinks. Some drinks are fortified with antioxidants, others with herbs. But the main components of a sports drink are always the same: sugar, salt, potassium, and water. Choose sports drinks with 5 to 8 percent carbohydrate. Studies show that this amount of sugar moves through your stomach and intestines fastest. To figure out the percentage of carbohydrate in a drink, divide the grams of carbohydrate per serving by the milliliters of drink per serving and then multiply by 100.

Energy bars. There are now more energy bars than I can keep track of, and it seems that each company has its own marketing gimmick. Some contain herbs, others vitamins. Some are kosher, others all-natural. Whatever the gimmick, look for a high-carbohydrate bar that contains 5 or fewer grams of fiber, 4 or fewer grams of fat, and 5 or fewer grams of protein. (The lower the fiber, fat, and protein, the better). Some bars are humongous, with 400 calories and nearly 100 whopping grams of carbohydrate. Other, mini bars contain only 100 calories and less than 25 grams of carbohydrate. You want to consume more than 100 calories (30 to 60 grams of carbohydrate) an hour, so look at the serving size and carbohydrate content on the label and eat accordingly. If your bar contains 25 grams of carbohydrate, you can eat the whole thing. If it contains 100 grams, you want to nibble on a quarter of the bar per hour as you exercise. And take frequent sips of water.

Energy gels. These puddinglike snacks come in small packages that you can easily store in a pocket or safety pin to your shorts or jersey. Most gel packets contain about 100 calories and 25 grams of carbohydrate. I suggest sucking down only half of the gel packet at a time, since some people complain of stomach upset when they consume the whole packet at once. And make sure to swallow generous gulps of water with the gel to move it through your stomach faster. Experiment with different brands and flavors to find the ones that are the least sticky, best tasting, and easiest to transport and open.

Old favorites. You can eat plenty of other regular foods during exercise, even though the companies that make them don't market them specifically to those of us who play hard. Here are some examples of snacks that are nearly 100 percent carbohydrate. Each of the following servings will net you 25 to 50 grams of carbohydrate per hour: fig bars (2 to 5 per hour), Twizzlers (one 2½-ounce package per hour), Gummi Bears (one to three handfuls per hour), jelly beans (10 to 30 per hour), and bananas (two per hour).

Electrolytes

Electrolytes are substances that regulate essential bodily functions, including heart rate, blood pressure, and nerve impulses. Sports drinks, energy bars, and other performance foods usually contain sodium, potassium, and sometimes other electrolytes such as calcium and magnesium. Most important for your fit body, sodium may improve your ability to absorb sugar and water, helping you stay fueled and hydrated.

You lose both sodium and small amounts of potassium when you sweat. Under most circumstances, you don't lose enough to make you deficient in either nutrient. But during an endurance effort such as a marathon, a century bike ride, or an adventure race on a hot and humid day, you can lose enough sodium to run dangerously low.

The condition is actually more common if you rely on water only to hydrate. Though dehydration is much more common, you can actually drink too much water, which dilutes the sodium levels in your blood, setting off an electrolyte imbalance and leading to a serious problem called hyponatremia. This condition can trigger seizures, coma, and even death. Initial warning signs include confusion and disorientation, muscle weakness, and vomiting.

Women and slower beginner endurance exercisers are most at risk. According to a study from the New Zealand Ironman Triathlon, 18 percent of the finishers were hyponatremic, with three times as many women suffering as men. In 73 percent of the cases, overconsumption of water was the culprit.

Fortunately, only ultra-endurance athletes need to worry about such complications. Most of the rest of us have more than enough salt in our bloodstreams from eating salt-rich processed foods. Still, the salt in a sports beverage does have a purpose—it helps your body retain water. It also makes you thirsty, which causes you to drink more. That means you're less likely to be dehydrated. It also means that you won't have to make frequent pit stops.

How much salt do you need? Look for beverages that contain 50 to 250 milligrams of sodium per serving. Most common sports drinks, including Gatorade, fit that description. As for potassium, most sports drinks contain only a small amount of this mineral because replacing it is not critical during exercise. You can easily replace any exercise-induced potassium losses after a workout by eating a banana, orange, baked potato, yogurt, or raisins. And if you compete in endurance events, consume some salty food such as fat-free potato chips or pretzels during your race.

How to Eat While Working Out

What you should eat during exercise depends on the kind of exercise you're doing. The livelier the sport, the more you must pay attention to how you eat. Here are some specific tips for some different types of hard play.

Running

Running is both intense and bouncy, which makes fueling during exercise difficult for many people. It also requires little in the way of equipment, which makes carrying food a slight logistical problem. Fortunately, there are several solutions. Here are some tips to help you master your eating technique.

Dress smart. There is a wide selection of sports apparel and accessories on the market that make it easier to eat on the run.

- Stylish shorts from Race Ready (and some other manufacturers) come with convenient pockets for easy storage of your energy gels and bars. You can find these shorts at most specialty running stores or online.
- Cycling jerseys have pockets in the back for easy storage of gels, bars, and even house keys. Be sure to look for a lightweight shirt, since cycling jerseys generally run a bit thicker to shield cyclists from ride-induced wind.
- A wide selection of versatile fanny packs provide expanded carrying capacity for those on the go. Specially designed hydration waist packs can tote and even deliver water and other fueling fluids. As for comfort, the Camelbak, Nathan, and Ultimate brands were given high marks during a *Runner's World* magazine test. You can find these waist packs online or at specialty running stores.

Stash your food. Some runners drive their intended course a few hours before a run to stash water and sports drink bottles along the way. Afterward, they drive the course again to pick up their trash. I know one runner who buries his water along a route every other week or so. The water stays cold, strangers can't steal or tamper with the bottles, and the drinks are conveniently there when needed. Just make sure that it's okay to bury your drinks in the spot you've chosen, and remember to pay attention to where you've buried them.

Choose your course. Some public parks offer convenient water fountains every mile or so. You can also stash some money in your shorts or tights and plan your route to pass by a convenience store where you can stop for water or sports drink.

Get friendly. If you run around your neighborhood, ask your neighbors to leave out water for you or allow you access to a garden hose.

Nibble slowly. When you run, your stomach bounces. The more weight you put into your stomach, the greater your chance of getting a side stitch or bellyache. Eat and drink only a little at a time but often, about every 15 minutes.

Choose liquids. Liquids move through your stomach quickest, so if you have trouble eating on the run, sports drinks should be your fuel of choice.

Cycling

The sport of cycling allows ample opportunity for transporting food. In addition to special jerseys that feature no-bounce pockets, the bike itself is equipped to carry easy-to-reach water bottles. And the absence of jostling allows you to eat more food without having to worry about side stitches. If you're a beginner, however, learning how to eat during a ride without swerving can be tricky. Here are a few pointers.

- Open your energy bars before you get on your bike. Put the bars in your jersey so that the open side is facing away from your sweaty back.
- Put easily grabbed foods such as raisins, fig bars, and crackers inside resealable plastic bags and store them in your jersey.
- Practice riding with your hands off the handlebar so that you can balance more easily when grabbing for food or your water bottle.
- Don't look down when you grab your water bottle. Keep your eyes on the road and use one hand to swat around until you feel the bottle. If you have trouble pulling and pushing the bottle back into its carrier, adjust the carrier at your next stop.
- Bring money with you so that you can buy food from a convenience store during the ride.

Swimming

Many swimmers believe that they don't need to hydrate because they're not sweating, but that couldn't be further from the truth. You do sweat during swimming; you just don't feel it. You need to hydrate just as often as for any other type of exercise.

But hydrating and fueling can be complicated. I'll admit that it's nearly impossible to eat and drink while you're swimming. So you have only one option: Take breaks. Keep a bottle filled with sports drink on the side of the pool and sip from it between laps. For me, sports drink is the only thing I can stomach during swimming. Any type of solid food gives me side stitches. Try to sip some sports drink after a sprinting interval set or every 20 or so laps. You don't want to wait until you have to take huge gulps because that's when you get a side stitch.

Hiking

Unless you're racing to the top of a mountain, hiking usually provides a low-intensity workout. You can pretty much break all the rules (like eating lots of fat or protein) and still make it to the top. Your muscles are not pulling that much blood away from your stomach, so your digestion isn't as impaired.

My Food Diary

Because I swim and run for less than an hour at a time, I don't have to worry about fueling. But cycling is another story. I'll go out with my training partners for 4-hour-plus rides. When I first started doing these long rides, I would feel great during the first half and then lose it during the second half. But I haven't bonked since I refined my eating down to a science.

I consume 100 to 140 calories every half-hour, starting 30 minutes into the ride. My food of choice is chocolate Gu. I also take along a bottle of sports drink and some sports drink powder. Once I finish the sports drink, I find some water, fill up the bottle, dump in the powder, and shake. I usually stop at a convenience store during the ride to stock up on more sports drink if needed. During really long rides, I bring along some low-fat potato chips and munch on them for extra salt.

Still, you do want to pay attention to how much your food weighs. If you'll be on the mountain all day, you need a huge amount of food and water, especially if the weather is hot. The problem is that the water will weigh you down. To lighten the load and hike in greater comfort, buy a large water pack that contains a plastic bladder. The clever design eliminates the struggle with heavy and unwieldy water bottles. And while it might seem like fun to share a bottle of wine and canned sardines at the summit, I can guarantee that at some point you'll regret toting something that heavy all the way up a mountain and then back down.

Your food will get jostled in your backpack, so opt for items that won't get smashed easily. Energy bars and trail mix survive much better than muffins and sandwiches.

Eat Smart
after Exercise

I f you eat the wrong food (or no food at all) after your exercise session, you'll drag around for the rest of the day with a headache and little energy. Your legs will burn walking up even a small flight of stairs. And when it's time to work out the next day, you'll find other, more sedentary things to do, such as taking a nap. Eat the right foods, however, and you'll feel awake and energetic. You'll burn even more calories because your metabolism will continue to run strong. And you'll have fresh legs and the motivation you need to exercise the next day.

Eating after exercise won't counteract all the calories you just burned, and you're going to eat another meal at some point in the day anyway. Having that meal right after your workout does the most good, and it will prevent you from bingeing on fats and sweets later. For optimum recovery, include these four essential elements in your Eat Smart diet plan.

1. **Fluids.** In addition to replacing what you sweated off during your workout, drinking copious amounts of liquid shuttles energy to your muscles and removes waste products.
2. **Carbohydrate.** Carbohydrate goes straight to the glycogen stores in your muscles, which speeds recovery from exercise. In fact, according to a study from Loughborough University in England, eating

workout q&a

Q: After a tough workout, I like to kick back with a few beers, but my buddies tell me that alcohol slows recovery. Isn't there any way I can recover and have my beer, too?

A: I certainly don't recommend drinking beer after a hard, sweaty workout, but I know that you probably drink it anyway. Just remember that alcohol slows your recovery by delaying rehydration and preventing carbohydrate from getting to your muscles.

That said, you can have a couple of beers if you drink intelligently. First, drink a bottle or two of sports drink until you're hydrated (your urine will be pale yellow to clear). Don't even think about having a beer until you've urinated at least once after your workout. Then, have your beer, along with some high-carbohydrate food such as pretzels. Alternate your beer with water or sports drink, and stop at two unless you're prepared to skip your workout the next day.

soon after a workout allows you to increase your exercise intensity the very next day. Researchers asked athletes to run on treadmills until they were so tired that they couldn't run anymore. They fed the runners about 600 grams of carbohydrate over the next 22 hours. The runners then got back on their treadmills and ran until they hit fatigue. The athletes ran significantly longer than when they consumed a medium-carbohydrate diet of only 400 grams between efforts.

3. **Protein.** You need this important macronutrient to repair muscle damage, boost immunity, and escort carbohydrate to your muscles.

4. **Antioxidants.** When you exercise to exhaustion by hiking all day, running for more than an hour, or cycling 50 or more miles, you breathe lots of oxygen. While necessary for life, oxygen is an unstable molecule. Once inside your body, it can change form and oxidize other molecules and cells, which damages tissues. In the short term, this is felt as muscle soreness. In the long term, it can contribute to

heart disease and cancer. Fortunately, antioxidants, which are found abundantly in fruits, vegetables, legumes, and whole grains, fend off oxidation and protect your cells from damage.

It's important to eat the right foods at the right times. The longer you wait to refuel, the less your body will benefit.

The First 30 Minutes

You need to consume calories and fluids as soon as you finish your workout. If you don't take in some carbohydrate during the first half-hour after you exercise, you may as well kiss your chances of having a good workout the next day goodbye.

But like most people, you may not feel hungry right after working out. Exercise drains blood from your stomach and intestines and moves it to your muscles. Without brisk bloodflow, your intestines don't receive enough oxygen to absorb and transport nutrients quickly and your digestive system "goes to sleep." For many people, however, the thought of eating after a workout makes them nauseated. Others simply want to shower and get dressed before thinking about food.

That's okay. You don't need a gourmet dinner immediately following your workout; you just need a quick snack of 100 to 400 calories, so down two glasses of a caloric beverage such as sports drink, milk, or orange juice. Stay away from caffeinated beverages, which tend to increase urine output, and carbonated beverages, which take longer to drink. On a hot summer day, consider having an ice pop or cold smoothie, especially if you're overheated and don't feel hungry.

Your Real Meal

After you've showered and dressed, eat a real meal of breakfast, lunch, or dinner, depending on the time of day. The amount you should eat depends on your weight, your gender, and the duration of your workout. But what you need to eat stays the same.

For many years, scientists thought that our nutritional requirements after exercise were much the same as those before and during exercise: carbohydrate, carbohydrate, and more carbohydrate. But after feeding people many different combinations of protein, carbohydrate, and fat, re-

Recipe Revver ────────────

Chocolate Calcium-Blast Milkshake
Serves 2

When I was in high school, Mom didn't let me or my siblings eat much chocolate, so they often were jealous when Mom let me make and drink huge milkshakes after track practice. As always, Mom knew best; I *needed* the calories and the protein. Since then, I've developed a more healthful version of my favorite chocolate shake.

    5 ice cubes
    ¾ cup light vanilla ice cream
    2 tablespoons chocolate syrup
    ¾ cup fat-free milk
    ¼ cup nonfat dry milk

In a blender, combine the ice cubes, ice cream, syrup, milk, and dry milk. Process for 1 minute or until smooth, making sure that the dry milk is distributed evenly and is not stuck to the walls of the blender. (If it is, turn off the blender and use a spatula to scrape the sides, then blend again.) Pour into two glasses and drink immediately.

Per serving: *192 calories, 10 g protein, 34 g carbohydrate, 3 g total fat, 2 g saturated fat, 11 mg cholesterol, 1 g dietary fiber, 182 mg sodium*

searchers learned that a dose of carbohydrate and protein together works best. (Fat slows digestion and should be avoided immediately after exercise.) The study showed that including protein with carbohydrate in that first meal following exercise replenishes your glycogen stores faster than eating carbohydrate alone. Here's why.

You need protein to rebuild your muscles. After your workout, the individual amino acids that make up protein go to work repairing the damage you may have inflicted during your workout. They also help shuttle carbohydrate and fluids to your muscles and other parts of your body. Some amino acids even seem to boost your immunity levels.

Carbohydrate provides fuel. Eating lots of carbohydrate is the fastest way to refill your gas tank for your next workout. You want potatoes, rice, soda, sports drink, licorice, raisins, bread, and other starchy, sugary foods that get carbohydrate into your system quickly.

According to one study, the optimum ratio is about 3 grams of carbohydrate to 1 gram of protein. For example, a postrace meal of cereal with milk, or rice with a small portion of chicken provides the right combination of carbohydrate and protein.

To eat smart after exercise, you also need plenty of fluids—about 16 ounces for every pound of sweat you lose. You can gauge how much you've sweated by weighing yourself before and after you exercise. If that's too much trouble, monitor your urine color. Drink plenty of fluids until your urine is pale yellow to clear.

12 Real Meals for Refueling

During your first real meal, your body needs at least 400 calories of both carbohydrate and protein to replenish your glycogen stores. If that meal is also rich in antioxidants, you may fend off muscle soreness as well. Here are 12 quick and easy, antioxidant-packed, postexercise favorites. Some of these meals are mini meals—they're relatively low in calories and are geared toward smaller women whose exercise sessions are light to moderate. Others provide more fuel for women and men who play long and hard. All of the meals contain the right combination of carbohydrate and protein.

- ⅓ cup each soy nuts, dried papaya, and dried peaches and 8 ounces cranberry juice

My Food Diary

I don't have time to come home from a long bike ride, plop on the couch, and nibble for the rest of the afternoon; I head back to work. I used to just have a bagel or whatever I could find and then feel lousy both at work and during my workout the next day because I wasn't eating enough calories or enough protein. Now I know better, so I usually eat one of the following quick-and-easy meals for the nutrients I need.

- A Chocolate Calcium-Blast Milkshake
- A tuna sandwich on large pieces of bread
- A bottle of sports drink, which supplies 400 calories of carbohydrate and protein

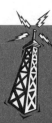

Nutrition News Flash

I love to swim, so I enjoy putting to rest the myth that swimming makes you hungry. Many people tell me that they avoid swimming as a form of exercise because of the post-pool cravings. But swimmers don't need to eat any more food after a workout than runners, walkers, or cyclists.

Researchers from the University of Toledo in Ohio asked a group of triathletes to either swim or run for 45 minutes. Then they escorted both groups of people to a room full of food and watched what the athletes ate during the next 2 hours. Both the swimmers and the runners ate the same amount of food, and both rated their hunger levels about the same.

- ½ cup frozen blueberries swirled into 1 cup low-fat lemon yogurt and a one-serving package of wheat crackers
- One nutrient-fortified energy bar containing 8 to 10 grams protein and 8 ounces low-fat milk or soy milk
- One small microwaveable bean burrito with 4 tablespoons bottled salsa and a small can of orange juice
- Two mozzarella cheese sticks, a toasted whole grain English muffin, and an orange
- A fruit smoothie made with soy milk, fruit, and frozen yogurt
- 6 ounces fruit-flavored yogurt with a handful of cashews and half a bagel
- A tuna sandwich on large pieces of sourdough bread
- Cheese sandwich and fruit salad tossed with walnuts
- Low-fat cottage cheese with sliced fruit
- A couple of cubes of low-fat Cheddar cheese and an apple
- Three rice cakes smeared with peanut butter and a glass of orange juice

Refueling after Longer Efforts

After an all-day hike, a long bike ride, or other endurance effort, you need more than one meal. Follow your initial 400-calorie meal with high-carbohydrate foods every 2 to 4 hours. Good choices include bread, beans, vegetables, fruit, pasta, potatoes, and rice. Don't forget to replenish your fluids by drinking frequently.

Following a long workout, you should consume 600 grams (or 2,400 calories) of carbohydrate in the next 24 hours. Try to average 50 grams every 2 hours.

Fueling for
Special Situations

Eating smart is not a one-size-fits-all phenomenon. "Smart" depends on your goals, your lifestyle, and your personal needs. There are numerous goals for eating smart, but there are two special situations that can turn smart eating on its head: vegetarianism and pregnancy.

I'm probably asked more questions about these topics than about any other. That's because they both put unique demands on your Play Hard eating plan. For example, a vegetarian lifestyle, while definitely a healthy one, can pose some challenges to playing hard. And pregnancy brings on a host of changes and a need for more calories, more of certain nutrients, and more fluids. Here's a look at the eat-smart plan for each of these situations.

Vegetarian Eating

Choosing to go vegetarian is a healthy decision. Vegetarians tend to have lower body mass indexes, lower cancer rates, lower total cholesterol levels, and lower LDL (bad) cholesterol levels than meat eaters. They also tend to live longer because vegetarian diets tend to be high in fiber, low in fat, and loaded with antioxidants and phytochemicals.

But getting all of the different nutrients that your body needs can be challenging, especially if you exercise on a regular basis. You must make

Recipe Revver

Tempeh–Snow Pea Noodle Salad
Serves 5

The following recipe satisfies 20 percent of your iron needs, 6 percent of your daily calcium needs, and 212 percent of your needs for vitamin C.

1 package (8 ounces) soba noodles
1 package (8 ounces) tempeh, diced into small pieces
2 cups snow peas, cleaned
1 cup sliced water chestnuts
1 teaspoon sesame oil
1 bunch scallions, chopped
4 tablespoons light soy sauce
¼ cup sweet rice wine vinegar
   Juice of 1 lemon
4 teaspoons sesame seeds

In a pot of boiling water, cook the noodles according to the package directions. (They cook quickly, in about 4 minutes.) When done, rinse the noodles under cold water and drain. In a large bowl, toss the noodles with the tempeh, peas, chestnuts, oil, scallions, soy sauce, vinegar, lemon juice, and sesame seeds. Cover and refrigerate for 1 hour before serving.

Per serving: 322 calories, 16 g protein, 53 g carbohydrate, 5 g total fat, less than 1 g saturated fat, 0 mg cholesterol, 5 g dietary fiber, 1,121 mg sodium

up for the nutrients that nonvegetarians get from eating meat. With the right food combinations, the holes in your diet can be patched, but for the list of nutrients that follows, the fixes can be tricky.

Protein. With the exception of soybeans, no single vegetable or grain provides all of the essential amino acids that your body needs. If you eat dairy products and eggs, those animal sources will provide the amino acids you need to make new proteins in your body. If you don't, then you must combine the right vegetables and legumes with the right grains.

You need 60 to 100 grams of protein a day. The standard 3-ounce serving of lean beef provides 21 grams. To get that amount of protein as a vegetarian, you must eat legumes and grains together. For example, 1 cup of curried chickpeas mixed with 1 cup of rice would amount to 21 grams of complete protein. So does a square of cornbread topped with 1 cup of cooked pinto beans.

Eat these complementary protein foods at the same meal if possible. It's okay to eat an occasional meal of incomplete protein as long as you eat the complementary protein a few hours later or at your next meal. Eating 1 cup of cooked beans along with approximately 1⅓ cups of cooked grain will provide the essential amino acids in the proper proportions.

Tofu and other soy products are an exception. Technically a legume, soybeans are in a class all their own. Ounce for ounce, soy protein is just as good as milk or meat when it comes to supplying quality protein and amino acids. In other words, there's no need to combine foods.

There's another reason to make soybeans a regular part of your eating plan. Several studies show that soybeans can help protect you against cancer and heart disease and may even curtail menopausal symptoms. Researchers believe that the phytochemicals in soybeans, especially one called genistein, act as antioxidants, which can slow the progression of aging.

Calories. Consuming enough calories is important for vegetarians who play hard. A vegan, or totally vegetarian diet, is higher in bulk than a diet that contains meat and dairy, but it does not contain as many calories as a diet that includes meat and dairy, so you may end up eating more food but consuming fewer calories. If you need 3,000-plus calories a day, salads just won't cut it. Try eating more whole grain cereal and bread, beans, nuts, and seeds. Peanut butter and crackers, for example, have protein as well as a heavy dose of calories.

Keep in mind, however, that if you do drink milk, you can easily overdose on calories by eating high-fat cheeses, eggs, and milk. Choose low-fat and fat-free versions of these dairy products when possible. And watch out for animal fats added to processed foods.

Vitamin B$_{12}$. You need only a millionth of a gram a day to keep blood cells healthy and to maintain the covering around nerve fibers, but B$_{12}$ is found exclusively in animal products. Going without it is not an option because a deficiency contributes to heart disease and can eventually result in spinal cord degeneration.

If you drink milk and eat eggs, you're fine. If you are a vegan, you have to eat B_{12}-fortified foods such as soy milk or cereal, or you must take a supplement to get enough of this vitamin. Gravitate toward fermented vegetable products such as miso and tempeh, which contain vitamin B_{12}.

Calcium. You need calcium for bone strength, cancer prevention, and blood pressure regulation, among other things. If you consume two to three servings of milk and other dairy products a day, you're getting all the calcium you need. If you don't drink milk, however, you're probably deficient, at least by Western standards. I say that because some believe that vegetarians don't need to consume as much calcium as those who eat meat. The theory is that vegetarians don't eat as much excess salt and protein as meat eaters, and this protects the calcium stores in their bodies.

More research is needed to determine whether this theory is true, so for now, I suggest that you bone up on calcium. After all, you don't want to find out that you could have avoided osteoporosis by eating more calcium when you were younger.

If you're a vegan, eat two servings daily of dark green, leafy vegetables such as collards, kale, turnip greens, and mustard greens. Eat generous amounts of legumes, tofu, quinoa and buckwheat, nuts, and seeds. Use blackstrap molasses in the doughs and batters of breads, muffins, and other baked items to increase the calcium content. And drink calcium-fortified soy milk.

Iron. You need iron to develop hemoglobin, which carries oxygen from your lungs to the rest of your body. Beef is your all-around best source of absorbable iron. While vegetables, whole grains, and legumes all contain some iron, your body doesn't absorb it as well.

If you're a woman, you need to make a special effort to eat foods high in iron, including green, leafy vegetables that are low in oxalic acid, which blocks iron from getting into your bloodstream. Including vitamin C–rich foods in your meals will increase your iron absorption. You can get a good dose of iron from lentils, kale, collard greens, dried fruit, and fortified breakfast cereal. Eat two servings of iron-rich foods a day.

Zinc. Meat is the major source of zinc, which plays a huge role in maintaining your health and your energy level. The high amounts of fiber in your vegetarian diet will bind to some of the zinc in your digestive tract, preventing absorption. To get enough zinc, eat several servings of wheat germ; whole grains; dried yeast; pumpkin; sunflower seeds; dark, leafy greens; miso; and fortified breakfast cereals each day.

All totaled, to get the nutrients you need, you should eat two daily servings of greens, eight servings of whole grains, and two servings of seeds or legumes.

Quick and Easy Tips

Getting all of the nutrients you need into your body doesn't have to be a chore. You can easily work them into your diet without measuring, counting, and sizing up your food. Here are some suggestions.

- Add beans to just about every dish you make, including soups, salads, casseroles, and brown rice. Combine them with grains for complete protein. Beans provide protein, fiber, iron, zinc, folate and other B vitamins, and potassium.
- Always go whole. You'll get more nutrients from whole grain foods than from refined grain products. So use brown rice, whole wheat pasta, and whole wheat bread, and try new grains such as quinoa, barley, oats, and amaranth. Quinoa is a power grain that contains a healthy dose of protein.
- Limit your consumption of junk foods such as candy and other sweets that contribute little or no nutritional value to your diet.
- Try soy substitutes. These days, you can find soy made into just about every food you can think of, from butter to cheese to sausage to hot dogs. And there are always the old standbys of tofu, tempeh, and miso. Eat soy nuts as a snack, and try soy butter and soy cheese. All of these products contain a wealth of important nutrients, and most of them are fortified with the nutrients that vegetarians need most. Try to eat 25 grams of soy protein a day, which is the amount in two garden burgers.
- Use packaged mixes. I love a line of products called Tofu Classics; the dishes are tasty, low in fat, and loaded with protein and fiber. Then there are the just-add-water products: Put them in a

Eating Smart for...
Vegetarians

To get all of the nutrients you need from nonmeat sources, just follow this food plan.

Breakfast
 1½ cups nine-grain cooked cereal topped with 1 ounce chopped almonds
 ¾ cup blueberries
 2 tablespoons honey
 8 ounces soy milk

Morning Snack
 2 ounces trail mix (raisins, dried papaya, pumpkin seeds)

Lunch
 One bean burrito (1 cup black beans, ½ cup rice, 1 ounce soy cheese)
 ¼ cup salsa
 1 cup fruit salad

Afternoon Snack
 One banana spread with 2 tablespoons peanut butter
 8 ounces cranberry juice

Dinner
 Spinach pasta with "meat" sauce (1 cup spinach pasta, ¾ cup red sauce, two (soy) veggie
   burgers crumbled into sauce)
 1 cup steamed broccoli
 1½ cup dark greens tossed with 1 tablespoon olive oil vinaigrette
 1 ounce dark chocolate

Calories: 2,500; Protein: 92 grams; Carbohydrate: 413 grams; Fat: 26% calories

saucepan, add water, and presto—you have a bean curry or couscous with lentils.

Eating for Pregnancy

You'll be happy to know that staying fit is good for both you and your
baby. Obstetricians used to warn pregnant women against exercise, fearing
that the heat or high heart rate would harm the fetus. Plenty of women lis-

tened and felt stressed, tense, and fat throughout their pregnancies.

Doctors now say that women who don't exercise may be doing their babies and themselves a disservice. Numerous studies show that fit moms have healthier pregnancies, easier deliveries, and smarter and healthier babies. Even after labor and delivery, moms who exercise burn off the fat from their pregnancies faster and experience less postpartum depression. And research shows that a sedentary woman can actually begin an exercise program during pregnancy as long as she keeps her intensity low and stops after 20 to 30 minutes.

You do still need to take some nutritional and physical precautions. Pregnancy brings a wide array of physical changes over the course of your 9-month journey. Plan on gaining 20 to 30 pounds, including a blood volume increase of a staggering 50 percent; extra breast, uterine, and fat tissue; and the baby itself.

Nutrition News Flash

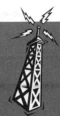

A review of all the available research reveals that exercising during pregnancy provided the following beneficial effects for Mom: improved mental well-being, limited weight gain, easier labor, a faster recovery from childbirth, and improved fitness. The studies also found that the baby of an exercising mother was born with less body fat, an improved tolerance for stress, and advanced brain and nerve maturity.

Gaining this weight sensibly requires smart eating, especially if you plan to exercise during pregnancy. Be sure to talk with your obstetrician about the types of activities that are most conducive to your changing center of gravity and larger size, such as swimming, walking, and recumbent stationary cycling. Your doctor should also inform you about limiting the intensity of your exercise and monitoring your heart rate during activity. Finally, avoid drastic elevations of body temperature, such as those caused by exercising in the heat or working out too long or too hard because too much heat really may harm the baby. Fortunately, your own fitness and your pregnancy improve your ability to dissipate heat, provided that you are adequately hydrated.

Your body and baby need extra calories, extra protein, and an array of vitamins and minerals to support both pregnancy and exercise. Here is what you need and how to get it.

Eating Smart for...

Pregnancy

I'm only 5'2", and my tummy started growing early during my pregnancies, which meant that I had little room for my stomach to expand during eating. This resulted in horrendous indigestion following meals and left me feeling unable to do my daily swim or bike ride. I had to completely change my eating strategy from eating about 4 meals daily to eating 8 to 10 times per day. Here's the plan I followed.

Morning

1 cup oatmeal with 1 tablespoon honey and 2 tablespoons raisins and almonds

8 ounces fat-free milk over 1 cup fresh blueberries

One mozzarella cheese stick with ¼ cup dried fruit trail mix (dried mango, apricots, raisins) with soy nuts

Midday

½ tuna sandwich on whole grain bread, topped with tomato slices

One apple with 2 tablespoons peanut butter

1 cup yogurt with ½ banana, sliced

Two small wheat crackers spread with 1 tablespoon hummus

Evening

One soy burger on whole wheat bun, topped with 2 tablespoons corn salsa

½ cup frozen yogurt with 1 tablespoon chopped almonds

Calories: 2,000; Protein: 85 grams; Carbohydrate: 270 grams; Fat: 30% calories

Protein. Being pregnant means that you need an additional 10 grams of protein each day. If you exercise, your protein needs increase even more, so add another 10 to 20 grams. Focus on quality protein sources such as soy, eggs, lean meats, fish, poultry, and beans and grains.

Calories. Pregnancy boosts your energy needs by 300 calories a day, sometimes more during the last several weeks of gestation. If you exercise, you need to eat additional calories to offset the calories burned during your activity so that you continue to put on needed weight and help your baby grow properly. Add 200 to 300 calories for each half-hour of moderate activity, such as walking or swimming.

Don't worry if you feel too sick to swallow that much food. During the first few months, when morning sickness is at its peak, the extra calories aren't as critical as they are during the second and third trimesters. If you're really nauseated, switch to a snacking lifestyle. Many pregnant women find that they can keep down smaller meals more easily than large ones.

Vitamins. Your prenatal multivitamin/mineral supplement should give you what you need, but be sure to eat at least five servings of fruits and vegetables each day for adequate vitamin intake and for the carbohydrate they provide to fuel your exercising muscles. Folate, a B vitamin that is especially crucial for your baby's healthy development, is found in citrus fruits, enriched grain products, and green, leafy vegetables. Your prenatal vitamin should include 400 micrograms of folate.

Calcium. Include calcium-rich foods such as fortified soy milk and orange juice along with yogurt and other dairy products to ensure that you and your baby get the amount needed for healthy bones (and for milk production, if you plan to breastfeed). Be sure to consume three to four daily servings of high-calcium foods.

Iron. Your need for iron doubles to 30 milligrams a day to help manufacture more blood and to boost stores of iron that are transferred over to your baby during the last months of pregnancy. Your physician will undoubtedly recommend that you take a prenatal multivitamin/mineral supplement to cover this increase. Be sure to eat good sources of iron such as fortified breakfast cereal, lean meats, beans, and wheat germ.

Carbohydrate. Regular exercise increases your need for carbohydrate. If you aren't gaining enough weight, increase your servings of potatoes, grains, fruits, and vegetables.

Essential fats. Healthy fats from fish, nuts, and flaxseeds are vital in the development of your baby's brain and nervous system. Make sure you eat these foods on a regular basis.

Fluids. Fit women need extra fluids to replace the sweat lost during exercise. Pregnant and lactating women need even more. You should drink *at least* eight 8-ounce glasses a day. When you're pregnant, dehydration may do more to you than give you a headache and make you feel lethargic; it can actually bring on premature labor, so don't skimp on the fluids. Your goal is urine so pale that you can't see it when you look in the toilet.

chapter seven

Eating to Overcome Fitness Barriers

An uncooperative body can easily destroy the best-laid fitness plans. Anything from persistent tummy aches to sore joints and muscles can force you to cut short an exercise session or not attempt one at all.

The unfortunate fact of becoming and staying fit is that sometimes it hurts. Increasing your mileage on the roads or trails and lifting heavier weights in the gym challenges your muscles and tendons in new ways, which is good. What's not so good is when those same muscles and tendons cramp up or feel sore.

While cramping and soreness both relay the same message of pain to your brain, they are really two different things. Cramps are brief, involuntary spasms in which the muscle contracts against your will. Muscle soreness can last for days and is usually a sign of small tears in your muscle.

Exercise can also do a number on your gastrointestinal (GI) tract. Problems arise because your stomach and GI tract are one sensitive system. Ask a little too much of this system and it throws a kind of "temper tantrum." During exercise, you may combine dehydration, heat, bouncing, and digestion. Any one of those elements may not tax your GI tract enough to make you take notice. But add two or three of them together and the result is diarrhea, heartburn, nausea, or side stitches.

That's because exercise diverts blood from your stomach and intestines to your working muscles, compromising your GI tract. During exercise, your intestines get little blood, oxygen, and fluid. When you are dehydrated, that compounds matters. The same is true for heat, which is often (but not always) a result of dehydration.

I feel especially sorry for those who experience GI woes because it's embarrassing to seek help. I get so many questions about bodily functions that I even have a name for them—FAEQs, or Frequently Asked Embarrassing Questions. Too often, people think that they are alone with these dilemmas. Ever so quietly, they whisper to me at race clinics when no one's around, "I often feel the urge to go, you know . . . uh . . . um . . . well . . . number two . . . when I'm exercising. Is there something wrong with me?" Or they slip notes to me after class: "I often pass gas during my yoga class. Please help me!" Or they send me a discreet e-mail: "I get heartburn during my swimming workout that really hurts; how can I make it stop?"

If people weren't so secretive about their GI problems, they'd find out that they have plenty of company. One study reveals that an estimated 30 to 50 percent of endurance runners experience some intestinal trouble, from cramping and nausea to bouts of flatulence and diarrhea during or after running. In short, GI problems are common during exercise.

Fortunately, you don't have to continue to be inconvenienced; these are all easily solved with smart eating. Here's how to beat each problem.

Muscle Cramps

Muscle cramps plague many fitness enthusiasts, especially during warm weather when they venture out into the heat more often. In fact, studies show that 30 to 50 percent of athletes who participate in endurance activities occasionally experience exercise-induced muscle cramps. These painful muscle spasms usually strike either during a long session of exercise or soon after you finish. Unfortunately, they often cut short workouts and keep some people from exercising altogether.

The cause of exercise-induced cramping has long been debated. For decades, researchers postulated that dehydration from heavy sweating on hot days and loss of electrolytes such as sodium and potassium were to blame for exercise-related cramping. This fluid-electrolyte theory is still

Eating Smart for...
A Day Free of Pain

Follow this menu to help prevent muscle soreness.

Breakfast
Antioxidant-packed smoothie (½ cup ice, 1 cup frozen blueberries, 4 ounces soy milk, 4 ounces orange juice, ½ cup vanilla yogurt, and 2 teaspoons honey)
One toasted whole grain bagel spread with 2 tablespoons raspberry jam

Morning Snack
One sliced kiwifruit with ½ cup fresh pineapple chunks

Lunch
One salmon salad sandwich (two slices whole oat bread, 3 ounces salmon mixed with 1 tablespoon fat-free mayonnaise, and two tomato slices)
Two fig bars
12 ounces iced green tea

Afternoon Snack
One orange
8 ounces sports drink

Dinner
1 cup black-bean chili over 1 cup brown rice with 2 tablespoons grated cheese
2 cups baby spinach with ¼ cup chopped red pepper and red onion
One 3-inch square whole corn cornbread with 2 teaspoons honey
Six chocolate-dipped strawberries

Calories: 2,250; Protein: 83 grams; Carbohydrate: 392 grams; Fat: 18% calories

popular, but new evidence challenges this belief, especially since many people experience cramps during exercise in cooler temperatures and without major losses of sweat or electrolytes.

New studies using a technique that measures electrical activity of muscles both during and after exercise reveal that muscle fatigue is the culprit behind cramping. Fatigue brings on a series of internal changes that cause your muscle to enter a state of enhanced excitability. It suddenly shortens, resulting in a painful muscle cramp. The muscle usually relaxes after 5 to 15 seconds, but passive stretching of the cramped muscle, such as extending your leg back when you have a calf cramp, will bring almost immediate relief because the stretch interrupts the excitability cycle and helps your muscle get some rest.

Warding off cramps in the first place involves keeping muscle fatigue at bay. Here are some training and eating strategies that will help you stay on track.

Stay fueled. Make sure you drink fluids and consume carbohydrate during workouts lasting 60 minutes or longer. Eating a banana, a handful of dried fruit, an energy bar, or an energy gel and drinking plenty of water during a workout will help delay muscle fatigue.

Be fit. Being well-conditioned for exercises such as long-distance running will ensure that you're not overtaxing your muscles. Work up to longer efforts by increasing your duration slowly. That will ease your muscles into performing well during longer efforts and help you avoid undue fatigue and possible cramping.

Get loose. Prepare your muscles, especially those involved in previous cramping episodes, with passive stretching before exercise, and introduce more stretching throughout your daily fitness routine.

Cut workouts short. If you are plagued with cramps during longer exercise efforts, shorten your workout intensity or duration until you're cramp-free. Then increase your distance or time slowly.

Muscle Soreness

When you challenge your body during exercise, you make small tears in your muscles. In theory, this is a good thing because these small tears encourage your muscles to grow so that they can handle your next effort with ease. But to repair these small tears, your immune system responds with inflammation. The swelling puts pressure on nearby nerves, causing you pain.

It's normal to have mild discomfort after a tough exercise session, but you don't have to grit your teeth through pain or skip your next workout because of it. Eating the right foods can help you get rid of the pain faster. Here are some tips to eat by.

Pump up your antioxidants. Found abundantly in fruits, vegetables, and whole grains, these little dynamos thwart free radical damage in your muscles, which is one of the causes of postexercise muscle pain. Eat 8 to 10 servings of fruits and vegetables a day (the more colorful and varied the better) and 6 or more servings of whole grains such as barley, millet, quinoa, and wheat.

Eat more fish. A type of oil found in fish, omega-3 fatty acids act as a natural anti-inflammatory; research shows that an omega-3 fatty acid supplement of 1 to 1½ grams a day may reduce muscle pain. Rather than taking supplements, which can be expensive, eat fish rich in omega-3's, like salmon, twice a week.

Pop some vitamin E. This powerful antioxidant may help protect you from the oxidative damage caused by endurance exercise. It would be great to be able to get all of the vitamin E you need from foods, but that's difficult to do. During periods of heavy training, look for a vitamin E supplement that contains no more than 400 IU. Take your supplement with a meal because your body needs a small amount of fat for optimal absorption.

Explore the world of herbs and supplements. Not much research has been done in this area, and I'm personally not a pill popper. Yet I know many hard-core athletes who swear that supplements such as St. John's wort; methylsulfonylmethane (MSM), a natural source of sulfur; and glucosamine help ease muscle, joint, and tendon soreness. Herbalists say that St. John's wort and MSM act as natural anti-inflammatories. Glucosamine is thought to work by producing substances in ligaments, tendons, and joint fluids called glycoproteins, which may speed healing. If you want to give these supplements a try, follow the package instructions. Consult your doctor first if you are already taking prescription medications.

Diarrhea

Known in the sports world as runner's trots, diarrhea is very common during and after exercise, especially after running. Half of all runners report that they've had the urge to have a bowel movement during or just after a run, according to surveys.

In addition to the stress it puts on your GI tract, running shakes your bowels, stimulating the peristalsis action that pushes stool along in your intestines. But runners aren't the only fitness enthusiasts who complain of embarrassing and inconvenient pit stops; just about any endurance exercise can bring on this problem.

To limit the number of stops you're forced to make, try the following tips.

Time your fiber consumption. Many people who make frequent pit stops during a workout are eating high-fiber diets full of fruits, vegetables, whole grains, and beans. Fiber adds bulk to your stool, making pit stops much more likely during your workout. Fiber is good for your health, so you don't want to eliminate it from your diet. Instead, I recommend a timing experiment. Eat your lowest-fiber meal just before your workout. And if you have an extra-long or intense session coming up, eat a low-fiber meal the day before as well. After your workout, load up on those healthful fruits and vegetables.

Try liquid meals. Meal-supplement and -replacement drinks such as Ensure and Carnation Instant Breakfast are digested quickly, so they won't tax your intestines as much as solid foods eaten a few hours before your workout will.

Relax after eating. Give yourself 2 to 4 hours to digest any pre-workout meal.

Go easy on the caffeine. Caffeine can irritate your intestines and speed up your bowels, so beware of energy gels that contain caffeine. While no research shows that these gels will trigger a bowel movement, plenty of fitness enthusiasts have told me that they do.

Avoid sugar substitutes. Ingredients such as sorbitol and mannitol, which are found in gums, candies, and many diet foods, can cause diarrhea.

My Food Diary

At one time, I could just about count on making at least one pit stop during my long early-morning runs. I would feel small rumblings in my lower abdomen and try to ignore them, but they would get stronger and then turn into cramps. At that moment, I knew I'd have to either find a bathroom or duck into the woods. I became so embarrassed that I stopped running with my friends. After a bit of experimenting, I realized that skipping my morning latte kept my intestines from overreacting to the 1-hour-plus jostling. I do miss my caffeine, but I feel great after a 10-minute warmup, and better yet, I don't have to plan my running route around bathroom access.

Eating Smart for...
A Day of Uninterrupted Hard Play

The day before an important race or exercise session, try the following meal plan to reduce your chances of having to make an embarrassing pit stop.

Breakfast
1 cup Wheat Chex cereal with 4 ounces fat-free milk
One apple spread with 2 tablespoons peanut butter
8 ounces grapefruit juice

Morning Snack
One banana

Lunch
One tuna salad sandwich (two slices oatmeal bread, 4 ounces tuna mixed with 1 tablespoon fat-free mayonnaise, and two tomato slices)
Two oatmeal cookies
8 ounces fat-free milk

Afternoon Snack
1 cup grapes
8 ounces sports drink

Dinner
One baked potato (no skin) topped with 3 tablespoons grated Cheddar cheese, ½ cup low-fat cottage cheese, and ½ cup steamed green beans
Two sourdough rolls spread with 2 teaspoons trans-free margarine and 2 tablespoons jelly
½ cup frozen yogurt drizzled with 2 tablespoons chocolate syrup

Calories: 2,400; Protein: 97 grams; Carbohydrate: 385 grams; Fat: 24% calories

Stay well-hydrated. Dehydration can cause diarrhea by starving your bowels of needed fluids. Your bowels respond by letting fluids pool in your intestines, which later comes out as diarrhea. Make an extra effort to drink up before and during your workout, especially in the summer. You should drink 4 ounces of fluid every 10 minutes.

Switch your workout time. If you usually exercise in the morning, try an afternoon or early evening workout to see if your bowel trouble subsides.

Beware of antibiotics. Many types of antibiotics can kill the beneficial bacteria that live in your digestive tract, which triggers a bout of diarrhea. Research shows that eating a daily serving of yogurt that contains live cultures will replace the friendly bacteria, allowing you to continue your fitness program.

Lay off the drugs. Avoid aspirin and other medications that may irritate your intestines.

Try an over-the-counter remedy. Any brand antidiarrhea medication may help. Take one or two tablets 1 hour before your workout.

On the Road

When you travel to a race away from home (especially if that race is in a different country), you're at risk for diarrhea from bacteria in the water or the food. To avoid traveler's diarrhea, try these tips.

- Drink bottled water (not tap water), and use bottled water when brushing your teeth.
- Ask for bottled drinks *without* ice cubes.
- Drink only pasteurized milk.
- When buying bottled drinks, inspect the seal to make sure that it hasn't been broken. In some poorer countries, merchants cut soda with water to increase their profits.
- Eat only raw fruits and vegetables that you can peel.
- Avoid raw meats such as sushi, oysters, and sashimi.
- Steer clear of lettuce and other greens, which are tough to clean well.
- Wash your hands often.

If you do end up with traveler's diarrhea, you can still race (although you probably won't race well). Try to let some of the diarrhea run through you, since your body is trying to rid itself of the germ that made it sick. At least 4 hours before your race, however, start taking an over-the-counter antidiarrhea medication. And during the entire ordeal, make sure to hydrate well. The best type of beverage to drink during a bout of diarrhea is a sports drink; if you can't find one, make your own by mixing 1 teaspoon of table salt with 8 teaspoons of sugar and 1 quart of bottled water. When you eat, focus on easily digestible foods such as bananas, rice, applesauce, and toast (the well-traveled BRAT diet). White rice may encourage your intestines to soak up excess fluid, drying up your diarrhea.

Heartburn

Fitness enthusiasts who experience heartburn often eat too soon before exercise. Exercise such as swimming and yoga may bring on heartburn because you're placed in a horizontal position, which allows stomach acid to creep back up into your esophagus. Other types of exercise, such as running, may cause heartburn by contracting your abdominal muscles, essentially pushing acid back up and out of your stomach.

Some experimentation in the timing and amount of food intake may solve your problem. If your heartburn continues even after you try the following tips, see your doctor; you may have gastrointestinal reflux disease, which requires medical attention.

Avoid common offenders. Coffee, alcohol, fatty and spicy foods, chocolate, and citrus fruits have all been associated with heartburn, so avoid these foods in the few hours before your workout. If you are a heavy coffee drinker, try cutting back for good.

Eat smaller meals. Large meals take up a lot of room in your stomach, forcing stomach acid up where it doesn't belong. Switch to a nibbling lifestyle and try to eat small meals before your workout.

Stay upright. You come home from a long workout, eat a huge meal, and then flop onto the couch. Your supine position encourages all of the stomach acid needed to digest that large meal to come up into your esophagus, resulting in heartburn. As a general rule, try to walk around or remain in an upright sitting position for a couple of hours after you eat. If you do get heartburn, drink a glass of milk or water to wash the acid back down into your stomach; the milk might also neutralize the acid.

Lay off the painkillers. Research indicates that there are more serious reasons why you shouldn't take aspirin or ibuprofen before or during exercise, including an increased risk of kidney and liver damage, but these common painkillers can also cause heartburn.

Nausea

When a fitness enthusiast becomes nauseated, it's often from exercising in the heat. If possible, train and compete when the temperature is less than 80°F. When the temperature soars above 90°F, consider exercising indoors. Try the following tips as well.

Eat small. Lots of small meals seem to cause less nausea than one or two large ones do, especially during races. Take small bites of an energy bar or small slurps of an energy gel.

Go liquid. Many people find that they can handle liquids more easily than solid foods.

Get the salt you need. If you drink too much water before and during an ultra-endurance event, you can dilute the sodium in your blood, which can make you feel nauseated. In these cases, sports drinks are your best bet because they contain sodium. And any meal (even though you don't feel like eating it) can help sometimes because it replaces lost salt.

Experiment. Try different brands of sports drinks, energy gels, and bars. Each product contains a different combination of sugars, and some of those sugars may work better for you than others. Experiment with the amount of carbohydrate that you consume. Some people find that eating a little less than the recommended amount of carbohydrate during a race or workout seems to help ease their symptoms.

Try ginger. If you feel nauseated after an endurance event, ingest some ginger. Real ginger ale (look for ginger listed as one of the ingredients) or a ginger tea made with ground gingerroot may help ease your nausea. Some people find that defizzed Coke helps, too.

Try acupressure. Press your thumb or index finger on the inside of your wrist about 2 inches away from your hand (there's a groove formed there by two tendons). Hold it for a minute or two.

Don't fight it. If your nausea won't let up, do what your body asks. Lean over and throw up—you'll feel much better.

Side Stitches

No one is exactly sure what causes side stitches, but the most common theory centers on bouncing. As you run or swim, you jostle your

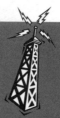

Nutrition News Flash

Many researchers suspect that jostling is the main cause of side stitches. But a study done by Darren Morton at the University of Newcastle in New South Wales, Australia, suggests that the cause may be more complex. Morton questioned hundreds of runners about their experiences with side stitches. Based on the answers, he concluded that at least some stitches are caused by the parietal peritoneum, a membrane that surrounds the abdominal cavity and is hypersensitive to movement. Morton also found that the following pre-exercise foods were most likely to cause side stitches: fruit (especially apples), fruit juice, chocolate, dairy products, and anything high in sugar or fat.

stomach and other internal organs. As they move around, they pull on the ligaments that hold them together. With enough pulling and pushing, these ligaments start to cramp, which is when you feel the pain in your side (or shoulder). To help put an end to side stitches, try the following strategies.

Eat and drink smart. Having too much weight in your stomach may cause it to push and pull against other organs, giving you pain in the side. Take small sips of your beverage and small nibbles of your food. And give yourself at least an hour between eating and working out, especially if your workout involves running or swimming.

Watch your sugar consumption. A type of sugar called fructose is not digested as quickly as sucrose and other sugars, and this may set off a side stitch. Avoid sports drinks that list fructose as the main sugar, and those with lots of sugar in general.

Learn how to breathe. Try getting rid of a stitch by breathing out forcefully and pushing your belly in at the same time. This will stretch out your diaphragm.

Chronic Problems

If you frequently have digestive problems during exercise and none of these tips help, see you doctor. You may have a serious underlying problem such as irritable bowel syndrome, an ulcer, or Crohn's disease. In those cases, avoid chocolate; caffeine; fatty, fried foods; acidic foods such as citrus fruits and tomato products; and extremely hot or cold beverages.

part two

Advances in
Fitness Eating

Power Foods

Look around the next time you're in the supermarket, and you'll see a growing selection of what I call designer foods: fruit juice fortified with calcium and beta-carotene, granola bars pumped up with antioxidants, and breakfast cereals stoked with fiber, just to name a few. Manufacturers have created these foods to meet consumer demand for better nutrition and good health. But before you stock your cupboards full of the latest designer fare, check out the superfoods that Mother Nature herself has to offer.

Many delicious natural foods pack whopping doses of vitamins, minerals, and fiber, just like their more expensive designer cousins. But unlike designer foods, natural whole foods contain potent doses of phytochemicals—substances that have been found to help fend off cancer, boost immunity, prevent heart disease, and speed recovery from a tough workout. Sure, manufacturers have tried to extract plant nutrients such as lycopene and insert them into designer food products. But the amounts they use are often not high enough to produce any effect. More important, research shows that it's the interaction of these nutrients in their natural states with other substances in your body that provides the most powerful performance benefits.

41 Superfoods for Power Eating

To perform at your peak in this fast-paced world, here are 41 super-foods—the best sources of fuel for your exercising body. Each is ready-made for optimum nutrition, providing the most bang for your nutritional buck. In addition to the best natural foods, which include whole fruits and vegetables, I've also added a few processed foods because every fit person will indulge in a quick snack once in a while, and it might as well be more nutritious than a candy bar.

Eat a wide variety of the power foods listed below on a regular basis, and you'll have more energy, strength, speed, and health than ever before.

Almonds

Because almonds are loaded with the antioxidant vitamin E, they can help reduce muscle damage and fend off age-related diseases. Almonds also give you a healthy dose of important minerals such as magnesium, iron, calcium, and potassium. Almonds do contain a hefty amount of fat, but it's mostly the monounsaturated type.

Eat almonds in a trail mix, sauté them into your next stir-fry, or just pop them in your mouth as a snack.

Asian Fish Sauce

Common in Asian stir-fry dishes and soups, this condiment made from ground-up fish is loaded with bone-building calcium. Just 2 table-spoons provides almost half of your recommended daily intake. And calcium is a valuable mineral for both women and men. Although osteo-porosis typically afflicts older women, doctors are finding more and more cases of bone loss among older men, which indicates that they didn't get enough calcium when they were younger. Besides building strong bones, optimal calcium consumption may fend off colon cancer, lower blood pressure, soothe premenstrual symptoms, and even encourage weight loss.

Fish sauce can be purchased at Asian groceries or specialty food shops, in the ethnic aisle of your supermarket, or online. Add a few tablespoons to your next stir-fry or soup. Because fish sauce contains a lot of sodium, however, use it moderately if you have a family history of high blood pressure.

Bagels

A bagel is an easy-to-eat snack that comes filled with muscle-fueling carbohydrate. Bagels truly are one of the best standbys before or after you exercise.

If you have a bagel before your workout, eat it either plain or with jelly or honey, but avoid fatty cream cheese, which slows digestion. Select whole grain bagels to get valuable fiber and other nutrients, including disease-fighting phytochemicals.

Bananas

Chock-full of carbohydrate and easy to digest, bananas are a classic superfood. They come with a nice dose of potassium, an important mineral that keeps blood pressure low. Bananas also supply plenty of vitamin B_6, which helps fuel your exercise.

Eat bananas alone, with peanut butter, or drizzled with honey, but eat them. Remember that you should be eating at least three servings of fruit a day.

Beans

If you're a vegetarian, black beans, lentils, chickpeas, and other beans are your best source of protein, iron, and soluble fiber. High in carbohydrate, beans are also loaded with folate (folic acid), which may fight heart disease and prevent birth defects during pregnancy.

Throw canned black beans, chickpeas, kidney beans, or any other type of bean in a blender with some spices to make a tasty sandwich spread, or add them to soups and salads.

Broccoli

Broccoli has it all. It's a great source of vitamin C, which may reduce exercise-induced muscle damage. It's also a good source of folate and the bone builders calcium and vitamin K. Broccoli is also chock-full of cancer-fighting phytochemicals called indoles.

Nutrition News Flash

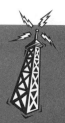

Fat has gotten a bad rap. Besides tasting great and helping you feel full, fat is just as important as vitamins and minerals. Special essential fats called omega-3 and omega-6 fats are crucial for a strong immune system and healthy skin and nerve fibers. Besides keeping you healthy, the right fats in the right amounts may even keep you exercising.

Researchers have long known that endurance training turns your muscles into better fat burners, and a number of studies done at the State University of New York at Buffalo suggest that a diet with 30 percent fat makes more sense for endurance exercise than one with less than 20 percent. In one of these studies, a group of runners who averaged 40-plus miles per week ate a diet with 17 percent fat for 4 weeks and then switched to a diet with 32 percent fat for another 4 weeks. At the end of each 4-week segment, the participants ran to exhaustion during a treadmill test. The men ran 24 percent longer and women 19 percent longer following the moderate-fat diet compared to the low-fat one.

Steam broccoli and squeeze some lemon over it, or chop it up and add it to your favorite pasta dish.

Brown Rice

All types of rice pack a powerful carbohydrate punch, but brown rice also provides a wealth of antioxidants. These will aid in your battle against heart disease as well as prevent exercise-induced muscle soreness.

Because brown rice takes 45 minutes or more to prepare, cook up a batch and freeze it. Immediately after a workout, you can simply add 2 tablespoons of liquid to a cup of frozen rice and cook it in the microwave. You can also buy instant, although it has slightly less fiber and nutrients than regular brown rice.

Canola Oil

Forget about all of those super low fat diets; they're for couch potatoes. People who exercise regularly *need* about 30 percent of their calories to come from fat. Of all the different sources of fat, canola oil is the best. Compared to other oils, canola has one of the lowest levels of artery-clogging saturated fat and one of the highest levels of monounsaturated fat, which lowers your risk of heart disease. Canola also supplies omega-3 fatty acids, which are found in fish and are known to fight heart disease.

Cereal

Packed with carbohydrate and fortified with vitamins and minerals, a bowl of cereal is a lot like a multivitamin but with much more fiber. Best of all, cereal takes only seconds to prepare and no time to clean up.

Eat cereal with 1% milk, or try mixing it with low-fat yogurt and fruit.

Chocolate

Nutritionists have long vilified chocolate because of its heavy dose of saturated fat as well as its sugar and overall calories. But the type of saturated fat found in chocolate isn't the same type of saturated fat found in butter and bacon. Chocolate's fat is called stearic acid and doesn't goo up arteries, thank goodness.

Even better, new evidence suggests that chocolate may prevent other foods from clogging up your blood vessels. That's because chocolate contains the same antioxidant nutrients that have made red wine famous for fighting heart disease. In fact, studies show that chocolate contains greater antioxidant properties than tea and even fruit such as blueberries. Cocoa powder, dark chocolate, and milk chocolate all contain respectable amounts of flavonoids, chemicals that prevent cholesterol-carrying LDL from oxidizing and damaging your arteries. The flavonoids in chocolate also help keep blood cells called platelets from sticking, lessening the risk of a clot that may cause a heart attack or stroke.

In fact, a 1-ounce square of dark chocolate has more flavonoids than a glass of red wine. And a cup of hot chocolate made with cocoa powder has about 75 percent the level of a glass of red wine, according to the research done by Andrew Waterhouse, Ph.D., and his coworkers in the enology department of the University of California at Davis.

So chocolate is definitely not as bad for you as was once thought. And although it's still high in calories, you have to splurge every once in a while to keep your diet interesting.

To avoid weight gain and satisfy your cravings, keep serving sizes small and reach for types of chocolate that have the most heart-healthy benefits. Eat no more than 1 to 2 ounces of chocolate a day and make it dark, since dark chocolate has more flavonoids than milk or white chocolate. For your daily chocolate dose, try my favorite super low fat chocolate boost: Blend 1 tablespoon of non-dutched cocoa powder with 2 table-spoons of hot water, then add 8 ounces of warm milk and a squeeze of honey for sweetness.

Clams

An excellent low-fat protein source, each 3-ounce serving of clams contains a whopping 24 milligrams of iron, enough to last you 2 days. Clams also supply a healthy amount of zinc, an immunity-boosting mineral that is notoriously low in many diets, especially those of people who exercise. If you're not consuming the 15 milligrams of zinc you need each day, your energy levels will stay low.

Drain and rinse canned clams, which actually have less fat and cholesterol than the steamed variety, and try adding them to spaghetti sauce.

Collard Greens

This green, leafy vegetable contains a cornucopia of vitamins, minerals, and phytochemicals that will boost your health and perhaps even preserve your vision. A recent study suggests that regular servings of collard greens and spinach can lower the risk of age-related degeneration of the retina. Researchers surveyed more than 800 adults on their vegetable and vitamin intakes and found that a weekly ½-cup serving of these greens cut the risk for eye disease by a third, and a 1-cup serving reduced risk by half. Researchers believe that carotenoids, a family of pigments found in vegetables and fruits, protect the eye from cell-destroying free radicals. Lutein and zeaxanthin, the carotenoids in collard greens, appear to have the most benefit. And there's more to collard greens than meets the eyes. They're packed with folate and vitamins A and C, plus calcium, magnesium, and potassium.

Add collard greens to your favorite soup, or toss them into a salad. Be sure to select fresh-looking leaves, and keep them in the refrigerator no longer than 5 days.

Energy Bars

Energy bars make great stand-ins for candy bars because they have almost none of the fat (1 to 4 grams in energy bars compared with more than 13 grams in many candy bars). What's more, most energy bars come fortified with 25 to 35 percent of the daily requirements of many vitamins and minerals—a benefit you would never get from a candy bar. Another advantage of an energy bar is its chewy texture, which allows it to last longer than a candy bar. And because of their high carbohydrate content, energy bars make good pre- and postworkout snacks.

I'll admit that an energy bar isn't often mistaken for a candy bar, but some of them taste surprisingly good. Try a few different brands to find the one you like best.

Fig Bars

These mini energy bars are great low-fat, high-carbohydrate snacks that satisfy your sweet tooth without packing fat into your arteries. Eat them right out of the package just before or after a workout, but don't get carried away.

Flaxseed

Sold as seeds, an oil, or a ground meal, flax contains high amounts of alpha-linolenic acid, a type of fat that can boost immunity, bloodflow, and possibly even endurance. Flax also keeps your platelets from clumping together and forming dangerous clots.

Use ground flaxseed when baking muffins. Buy breakfast cereals that contain flax (check the label), and mix flaxseed oil into your salad dressings. Store flaxseed in your refrigerator to keep it from turning rancid.

Garlic

Thanks to research, it's becoming clear that garlic wards off more than vampires. Garlic has been shown to lower blood cholesterol and may help prevent the formation of blood clots. It also lowers the risk of colon and stomach cancers; ongoing research suggests that garlic may lessen the chances of breast cancer. It's probably the phytochemicals allicin and S-allicysteine that are responsible for garlic's disease-fighting power. The two may work together to keep cancer-causing agents from latching on to cells.

To reap the most health benefits from garlic, slice it up and let it sit for 10 minutes before tossing it into your tomato sauce or stir-fry. While the chopped garlic sits, a chemical reaction takes place that prevents the high heat from destroying its healthful phytochemicals.

Ginger

Besides settling your stomach and working to reverse the effects of nausea, ginger may act as a natural anti-inflammatory, reducing joint and muscle pain. It also may prevent heart attacks by thinning your blood.

Look for dense roots. Grate the root into stir-fry dishes, cold salads, and fruit smoothies. Real ginger ale (look for ginger listed as one of the ingredients) and ginger tea are both made with ground gingerroot and can deliver some of the same healthful benefits.

Green and Black Tea

Green tea is an ancient and popular beverage that has long been thought to have health-promoting properties, and research findings indicate that its reputation is warranted. One study shows that green tea drinkers have a lower risk of cancer of the esophagus than nondrinkers. Another shows that it may protect against skin cancer. The protective agent in tea looks to be a substance called epigallocatechin gallate, or EGCG. It acts as an antioxidant, protecting cells from the damaging work of free radicals.

Black tea, made from the same leaves as green tea but blackened during the fermentation process, also contains EGCG. About 80 percent of the tea consumed worldwide is black tea, and although most research has focused on green tea, researchers suspect that black tea provides similar benefits. Black tea can be found anywhere—it's the kind Americans typically drink. Green tea used to be available strictly through specialty food shops or Asian grocery stores, but more and more it is finding a place on suburban supermarket shelves.

Try to drink one to two cups a day.

Kiwifruit

Tart and tasty kiwifruit is an excellent source of vitamin C. It's also high in potassium, which can help keep your blood pressure low. And remember, for the health benefits they provide, you should eat three to five servings of fruit each day.

A juicy kiwi makes the perfect postexercise snack on a hot day. The riper the fruit, the more satisfying it will be to your sweet tooth. Simply slice it in half and then use a small spoon to scoop the fruit from its peel. You can also mix it into fruit salads or your favorite fruit smoothies.

Lentils

One cup of cooked lentils contains 17 grams of protein, a whopping 8 grams of fiber—about one-third of the recommended Daily Value (DV)— more than 35 percent of your iron and potassium needs, and 175 percent of the Daily Value for the B vitamin folate. This last ingredient may be lentils' biggest contribution of all, as folate is crucial for the production of new cells, especially the millions of blood cells made daily. Plus, many of us don't get enough folate, especially pregnant women, whose need is greater.

Try lentils in casseroles, soups, and pasta or bean salads.

Milk

Drinking low-fat or fat-free milk is the easiest way to get high amounts of calcium into your body. Calcium is one of the more important nutrients for fit people because it aids crucial body functions such as bone-mineral formation, muscle contraction, and nerve conduction. Consuming adequate amounts of calcium helps prevent stress fractures, shinsplints, and possibly muscle cramps.

Milk makes a great postexercise recovery food because it provides both carbohydrate and protein.

Oatmeal

Oatmeal ranks as one of the best breakfast foods to eat if you're watching your weight because, as the saying goes, it sticks to your ribs. Oatmeal's high amount of water-soluble fiber does more than keep you full; it also lowers your blood cholesterol. High in muscle-fueling carbohydrate, oatmeal is a good source of iron.

Add dried or fresh fruit to your oatmeal for even more health power.

Oranges

Citrus fruit is nature's own sugary delight, bursting with natural sweetness and nutrients. The sweet taste of oranges comes from fructose, which is actually sweeter-tasting than table sugar. An excellent source of carbohydrate, oranges are full of vitamin C. This powerful antioxidant may help your muscles recover faster after exercise and will keep your immune system running strong. Oranges are also a great source of folate, which helps maintain optimal levels of hemoglobin for your oxygen-carrying red blood cells. The white pith on oranges is loaded with flavonoids that keep LDL (bad) cholesterol from damaging artery walls.

Oysters

The health titan of shellfish, just six oysters pack an amazing 500 percent of your DV for zinc, which is vital for building a healthy immune system as well as repairing and maintaining muscle tissue. Many endurance athletes are more susceptible to viral and bacterial infections after competitive events such as the marathon, which is why they need zinc; most people don't regularly meet the DV. And men, listen closely: Zinc is essential for sperm production and sexual functioning.

Add oysters to seafood stews or soups. A word to the wise: If you go out for oysters at an oyster bar, make sure it's a reputable establishment, since raw seafood can harbor parasites that cause illness.

Pasta

Famous as the quintessential carbo-loader, pasta is low in fat and is a great source of folate, which decreases your risk of heart disease. Pasta also serves as a great vehicle for other good-for-you foods such as tomato sauces, tofu, and clams. Use whole wheat pasta for an added dose of fiber.

Peanut Butter

Peanut butter is a good source of vitamin E, which is probably the most powerful antioxidant. The fats in peanut butter are mostly monounsaturated and polyunsaturated, which are the heart-healthy kinds.

Look for the natural form of peanut butter, sold in health food stores. It's a bit thicker than processed brands—you'll have to use some muscle power to stir it up—but it contains more healthy fats than many of the processed types. If you buy processed peanut butters, avoid those that list hydrogenated fats first on the list of ingredients.

Pretzels

Both hard and soft pretzels are high in carbohydrate and low in fat. Even salted pretzels are fine for those who don't have high blood pressure, as the sodium helps you retain the fluid you drink before and after exercise.

Pumpkin

You don't have to limit your pumpkin consumption to holiday pies. Pumpkin is so nutritious that you should eat it year-round in muffins, breads, and soups, or on its own, cooked with a little seasoning. Just a ½-cup serving packs more than 200 percent of your daily vitamin A needs (in the form of beta-carotene). Like its cousins, the butternut, hubbard, and other winter squashes, pumpkin contains several carotenes that all appear to have antioxidant properties. A ½-cup serving of pumpkin contains lots of fiber and about 10 percent of your daily needs for potassium, iron, and magnesium, all of which are crucial for muscle efficiency during exercise.

Whole pumpkin is easy to find during the fall and winter months, and you can prepare it simply by baking or microwaving pieces of it in a casserole dish until tender. Canned pumpkin is tasty and nutritious and can easily be stocked in your pantry year-round.

Raisins

High in carbohydrate and low in fat, this convenient snack supplies plenty of potassium as well as some iron. Like grapes, raisins also contain an abundance of heart-healthy phytochemicals.

The beauty of raisins is their easy-to-eat size. Stuff them into the pockets of your cycling or running jersey, or include them in a bag of trail mix for a healthy hiking snack.

Red Meat

Skimping on red meat in an effort to cut calories and fat can lead to iron deficiency, low energy levels, and poor exercise performance. Steak and other forms of beef are your best source of heme iron, the most absorbable form. More than half of the iron in beef comes from heme, compared with 40 percent in dark-meat chicken and 30 percent in white-meat poultry. Men need 10 milligrams of iron a day; women need 15 milligrams.

For a quick iron-rich meal, make fajitas with marinated flank or round steak, which tend to be lower in fat than other cuts. Chop up the steak with some tomatoes, onions, and peppers and toss them on the grill. If you don't eat beef, eat a food rich in vitamin C along with your fruits and vegetable sources of iron to aid absorption.

Salmon

Salmon and other types of "fatty" fish such as sardines are filled with omega-3 fatty acids, important oils that keep your immune system strong. They also may boost bloodflow, which could improve your workouts.

Many people don't get enough of these oils; research suggests that this deficiency may contribute to the development of heart disease and arthritis. In the human body, these fats transform into hormonelike substances that help regulate blood clotting and menstruation, among other things.

Make fish a regular part of your diet by eating two to three servings a week. Grill it and top it with a fruit salsa of sliced kiwi, papaya, cilantro, and a jalapeño pepper. The salsa adds important antioxidants as well as fiber.

Soup

A study at the University of Nebraska at Omaha found that vegetable-rich chicken soup helps halt neutrophils, the type of white blood cells in your immune system responsible for runny noses. Eating a bowl of chunky soup as your first course at lunch may also suppress your appetite for the rest of the day, according to several studies. Soup may also lower your calorie intake simply because it takes a long time to eat, which allows the relay system between your brain and stomach more time to transmit the "I'm full" message. And when made properly, soup is packed with an abundance of vitamins, minerals, phytochemicals, and fiber. In one hefty bowl of bean-and-barley soup, there's the same amount of protein as in a main entrée and two to three servings of vegetables. All of these nutrients work together to fight off heart disease and cancer.

Canned soups offer much of the same goodness as homemade, as long as you take the following precautions. Avoid cream soups or chowders, which usually contain too much fat. If you're watching your sodium intake, look for low-sodium varieties; check the label since many canned soups have 500 to 1,000 milligrams per serving (about one-third of your daily allotment). Look for soups that list 3 or more grams of fiber on the label.

Spinach

High in antioxidant carotenes, calcium, and iron, spinach is a true power food. The carotenes help ward off age-related diseases as well as protect your muscles from damage. The calcium keeps your bones strong, and the iron keeps your energy high.

Use spinach instead of iceberg lettuce to boost the nutritional punch of your salads. Also, sneak cooked spinach into lasagna and other casseroles. To increase iron absorption, make sure to eat something acidic or high in vitamin C, such as tomatoes or oranges, along with your spinach.

Strawberries

Strawberries (and many other berries) are low in fat and high in vitamins, especially beta-carotene, vitamin C, and folate. They also provide lots of fluid, making them a good snack after a workout, especially on hot days. Strawberries are loaded with ellagic acid, a powerful antioxidant that can inhibit tumor growth.

Mix strawberries with other berries in a fruit salad, or blend them with milk or yogurt for a nutritious postexercise smoothie. Or slice several juicy strawberries to put on top of your pancakes instead of maple syrup.

Sweet Potatoes

Sweet potatoes are full of carbohydrate, fiber, and carotenes, a family of antioxidants that prevents cancer.

(continued on page 88)

Build a Better Fruit Smoothie

One of the most powerful edibles around isn't a food but rather a number of foods. Smoothies are a blend of fruit, fruit juice, crushed ice, and milk, sorbet, or frozen yogurt. When blended, these foods give you all of the calcium, carbohydrate, protein, vitamins, minerals, and phytochemicals that you need in a meal. This powers your exercise, speeds your recovery, and helps keep you healthy.

There's a catch, though. Mix the wrong ingredients into your smoothie, and you end up with a glorified milkshake that's packed with unwanted calories and fat. Use the right ingredients, and you end up with a great-tasting, healthful treat.

Make sure your smoothie contains at least two different kinds of fruit and some fruit juice. Then add some crushed ice, nonfat frozen yogurt, sorbet, or nonfat ice cream. Mix in low-fat milk, soy milk, tofu, or plain yogurt for extra protein. For the best results, do it all in this order.

1. Put frozen ingredients (ice cubes, frozen fruit, sorbet) in the blender first. Make sure you keep these items golf ball–size or smaller so that they blend completely.
2. Add liquid ingredients and secure the blender lid.
3. Press the start button; blend on high speed for about 30 seconds.
4. Shut off the blender and open the lid. Add more liquid if needed. Free any chunks that are wedged on the bottom, put the lid back on, and blend for 30 more seconds.

To make your own signature smoothie, use my simple smoothie-making menu to mix and match your favorite ingredients. Start with about ½ cup of crushed ice or ice cubes; you can always add more if needed. Choose two fruits; use 4 ounces of juice; use ½ cup or more (to taste) of the frozen treats; add one of the optional protein ingredients if the smoothie is your entire meal; and select up to two of the optional flavorings and extras.

Fruit

One medium orange
½ banana
1 cup strawberries (fresh or frozen)
1 cup cubed cantaloupe
1 medium kiwifruit
¾ cup pineapple

1 cup blackberries (fresh or frozen)
1 cup raspberries (fresh or frozen)
1 cup sliced mango
1 cup cubed papaya
One medium peach
One medium nectarine

Juice

Orange
Grapefruit
Pineapple
Cranberry
Guava

Prune
Tomato
Carrot
Kiwi-strawberry

Frozen Treats

Fruit sorbet (strawberry, peach, mango, lime, or others)
Sherbet (orange, pineapple, berry, or others)

Nonfat frozen yogurt
Reduced-fat ice cream

Optional Protein

¾ cup plain, nonfat yogurt
6 ounces soy milk

6 ounces 1% milk
1 scoop soy protein powder

Optional Flavorings and Extras

1 teaspoon cocoa powder
1 tablespoon ground flaxseed (grind whole flaxseed in a coffee grinder)
2 tablespoons ground nuts such as almonds or walnuts
1 to 2 tablespoons powdered carbohydrate supplement

1 to 2 tablespoons wheat or oat bran (you'll need to add more liquid since these thicken your drink)
1 to 2 tablespoons peanut butter
½ teaspoon zest from an orange, lemon, or lime
Dash of vanilla, cinnamon, or nutmeg

Microwave the sweet potato until it's soft to the touch (about 4 minutes), split it open, and add a pinch of brown sugar and cinnamon plus a touch of butter or low-fat yogurt.

Sweet Red Peppers

These crunchy, colorful vegetables supply more immunity-boosting vitamin C than oranges. They're also loaded with carotenes.

Use red peppers as a colorful addition to any pasta dish or salad; also, cut them up and take them to work for a snack.

Tofu

Most vegetarians know that tofu is one of the best nonmeat protein sources. But even nonvegetarians should eat tofu regularly. Tofu supplies a decent dose of bone-building calcium and B vitamins. According to research, the soy protein found in tofu may help prevent cancer, heart disease, and osteoporosis. It may even decrease menopausal symptoms.

Like other soybean products, tofu contains isoflavones. These cancer-fighting substances have been shown to reduce the risk of prostate cancer in men and breast cancer in women. (The high consumption of soy products in Asian countries may be why the prostate cancer risk there is lower.) Genistein, an isoflavone found almost exclusively in soybeans, has been shown to block the growth of new blood vessels that feed cancerous tumors. This may eventually starve the cancer cells and inhibit tumor growth. Ongoing research is investigating whether purified genistein retains the same cancer-fighting properties as whole soybeans, or if other substances in soybeans work in tandem with genistein to fend off disease.

A 4-ounce serving of tofu contains 10 grams of protein (about 20 percent of your daily need) and more than 30 percent of the DV for calcium. Try tofu in stir-fries and soups, or marinate and grill it just as you would chicken. You'll normally find it refrigerated in the produce section of your grocery store.

Trail Mix

This favorite snack of backpackers is nutrient-rich and moderately low in fat if mixed wisely. Look for tropical versions of trail mix sold in bulk at grocery stores, or make your own with raisins, banana chips, dried pa-paya and apricots, and pumpkin and sunflower seeds. One ounce of this power mix has about 100 calories and is filled with potassium, iron, beta-carotene, and a small amount of fiber.

Since trail mix keeps well, you can always stash some in your workout bag, glove compartment, or office desk.

Turmeric

A colorful spice popular in Indian cuisine, turmeric is the major in-gredient in curry powder. Turmeric contains polyphenolic compounds that have antioxidant properties as well as some ability to fight inflammation in much the same way that aspirin does. Specifically, curcumin, a sub-stance found in turmeric, has been shown to inhibit inflammation and tissue damage. So plan an Indian meal after your next hard workout.

Add powdered turmeric to stews and casseroles for a lively flavor, or mix some into steamed rice for a colorful, high-carbohydrate dish.

Whole Grain Bread

High in carbohydrate, whole grain bread contains many of the same healthy phytochemicals as fruits and vegetables. Most whole grains also contain B vitamins, and some come with iron added.

Use whole grain bread for your sandwiches, or nibble on a slice be-fore or after your workout for a solid dose of fuel.

Yogurt

The word on yogurt is this: Two cups a day may keep colds and al-lergy symptoms away. A study from the University of California at Davis found that people who ate 2 cups of yogurt made with live bacteria cul-tures (specifically *Lactobacillus* and *Streptococcus thermophilus*) daily had fewer colds. Those with allergies experienced fewer symptoms. The theory is that the bacteria in the yogurt boosted the subjects' immune systems. Studies also show that these same bacteria may help women avoid vaginal yeast infections.

Yogurt is also a terrific source of muscle-fueling carbohydrate and pro-tein. And it contains more than 40 percent of the DV for calcium in a standard 8-ounce serving. Look for yogurt that says it contains live cultures, since pasteurization kills the bacteria.

Yogurt is perfect for a quick breakfast. Add fresh fruit and granola to plain nonfat yogurt to create a snack loaded with vitamin C, fiber, and other nutrients.

Maximizing the Power

As good as they are, your diet shouldn't revolve around these 41 power foods alone. Your body needs a wealth of phytochemicals, macronutrients, and micronutrients to fuel your exercise and your life. To determine if your body is getting everything it needs for maximum power, use the following list to see if your diet is varied enough. Simply check off the foods you eat during the next 3 days. The foods are grouped loosely (dairy, meats, vegetables). If you check off 28 or more foods, you're doing great.

❑ Cheese
❑ Eggs
❑ Ice cream and other dairy-based desserts
❑ Milk
❑ Yogurt
❑ Beef
❑ Fish
❑ Lamb, veal, and game
❑ Lunch meats
❑ Pork
❑ Poultry
❑ Beans and legumes
❑ Nuts and seeds
❑ Green, leafy vegetables
❑ Orange, yellow, and red vegetables
❑ Other vegetables
❑ Potatoes and other root vegetables

❑ Tomatoes and tomato products
❑ Berries
❑ Citrus fruit
❑ Fruit juice
❑ Melons
❑ Other fruit
❑ Bread
❑ Breakfast cereal
❑ Pasta
❑ Rice
❑ Whole grain products (quinoa, amaranth, couscous, barley)
❑ Cooking oil
❑ Margarine or butter
❑ Baked goods
❑ Candy
❑ Salty snacks
❑ Soft drinks

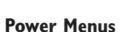

Power Menus

Knowing what you should eat is one thing; knowing when to eat it is another. Here are three performance menus for powering your day's hard play, based on the time of day that you exercise.

Morning Exercise

6:00 A.M.: Sports drink

6:20 A.M.: Workout

7:00 A.M.: Cereal with fruit and 1% milk

10:00 A.M.: Fig bar and a glass of water

Noon: Cold tofu salad and fruit salad from your local deli

6:00 P.M.: Pasta with clam sauce, a whole grain roll, a side of steamed broccoli, and a piece of chocolate for dessert

Afternoon Exercise

7:00 A.M.: Oatmeal with fruit, a side of yogurt with almonds sprinkled on top, and a glass of 1% milk

10:00 A.M.: Fig bar and a glass of water

Noon: Workout

1:00 P.M.: Sandwich with turkey breast, cranberry sauce, lettuce, and tomato on whole grain bread, served with a side of mixed fruit and some pretzels

7:00 P.M.: Grilled fish and a side salad

Evening Exercise

7:00 A.M.: Whole grain toast with peanut butter and a sliced banana on top, and a bowl of cereal with 1% milk

Noon: Beef-and-bean chili with cornbread

3:00 P.M.: Pretzels

5:30 P.M.: Workout

7:00 P.M.: Tofu, broccoli, and brown rice stir-fry with a sweet potato

chapter nine

New Fueling Products

During a run one day, my training partner, Terry, asked me, "What's the best refueling choice? Should I go with water, a sports drink, an energy gel, or an energy bar?" I knew I wouldn't be able to get away with a short answer. When it comes to performance nutrition, Terry always wants to know the whys, the whens, and the what-ifs. So we slowed our pace and spent the next hour discussing the nuances of fatigue and refueling.

Eating and drinking relieve the three main factors that cause fatigue: dehydration, or loss of fluids; lowered blood glucose; and depleted muscle glycogen. If you play hard, you can minimize the energy-depleting effects of your workout by refueling with a variety of cutting-edge products on the market.

As I told Terry, you have to use your own judgment about which products to try, then determine what works best for you. For workouts lasting less than an hour, water is adequate. (Just be sure to get a good dose of digestible carbohydrate 2 hours before your workout and within an hour afterward.) For workouts lasting longer than an hour, you'll need fluid and energy replacement. Energy bars, sports drinks, and energy gels are all effective energizers. Regardless of your choice, aim for 30 to 60 grams of carbohydrate per hour of exercise, which equals about 24 ounces of sports drink, two 1-ounce packets of energy gel, or one energy bar. Here is a closer look at the most popular new fueling products and how they can affect your performance.

Energy Bars

Serving size: One bar   **Calories:** 100 to 400   **Carbohydrate:** 20 to 50 grams
Extras: Vitamins, minerals, fiber, protein

Energy bars were born in the mid-1980s when Olympic Marathoner Brian Maxwell set out to develop a portable, solid, carbohydrate-packed fuel source for endurance athletes. Today, PowerBar, the original energy bar, is still the market leader, although countless other brands of energy bars have flooded the market in flavors ranging from cookies-and-cream to carrot cake to latte swirl. Many of these bars come packed with everything but the kitchen sink: protein, quick-release carbohydrate, slow-release carbohydrate, vitamins, minerals, and some extra ingredients for (according to label claims) burning body fat, calming nerves, and more.

Energy bars are a good, portable source of fuel for endurance exercise. And they can provide calories and nutrients during hurried days when you don't have time for a real meal. But the big question is whether you can digest them quickly enough during a moderate workout to reap the benefits. Is solid carbohydrate as helpful as liquid carbohydrate?

The answer is: probably. Several studies have shown that for a particular carbohydrate (glucose, for instance), it doesn't matter if it's in solid or liquid form, as long as you take it with enough water. It's readily absorbed either way.

Unfortunately, there has been far less research comparing different forms of carbohydrate (such as the sugar in a sports drink versus the oats in an energy bar) and the relative ability of each to maintain blood sugar levels during exercise. Two different kinds of carbohydrate may be digested at different rates and enter the bloodstream at different speeds. This rate of carbohydrate digestion and the subsequent appearance of sugar in the bloodstream is a food's glycemic index. A food with a high glycemic index (such as rice) is best during exercise, since it gives you quick energy that can be used immediately as fuel.

Because we don't know the glycemic indexes of various energy bars, you'll need to experiment to see which one works best for you. Also, many bars have added vitamins, minerals, fiber, or even fat and protein, some of which affect the glycemic index. It's not clear how much of a performance boost you can get from these extras, either.

What is clear is that when you eat an energy bar, you must drink water to help you replace fluids lost through sweat as well as to digest the bar. Some people find energy bars tough to get down during exercise, especially running, which is why finding a favorite brand with the right texture and taste for you is so important.

Energy Bar Rundown

Here is a roundup of some of the more well-known energy bars. Since so many companies make them, the bar you eat may not be on the list; in that case, check the label for nutrition facts.

Energy Bar	Size (g)	Calories	Carbohydrate (g)
Balance	50	200	22
Balanced Nutrition	50	190	24
Boulder Bar	71	190	37
Clif	68	250	42
EAS Protein	78	310	16
GeniSoy	62	230	31
Luna	48	180	25
Met-Rx	100	320	48
PowerBar	65	230	45
PowerBar Harvest	65	240	45
PR Bar	50	190	21
Tiger Sport	65	200	43
Twinlab Ironman	57	230	24

When choosing from the hundreds of bars out there, here are some characteristics to consider.

Calories. Most bars range from 100 to more than 400 calories. Before you grab a bar based on calories, check the label for the serving size. Some weigh a mere ounce (28 grams), while others are more than four times that size. And size becomes important when making bar-to-bar comparisons. Aim for 120 to 300 calories per hour of exercise.

Protein. During exercise, opt for bars with no more than 10 grams of protein (the amount in a glass of milk). Any more may slow digestion and the speed at which the carbohydrate travels to your exercising muscles.

Fiber (g)	Protein (g)	Fat (g)	Vitamins and Minerals (% Daily Value)
1	15	6	25–210
0	14	4	15–25
4	8	2	N/A
5	9	5	some bars fortified with antioxidants
1	33	7	25–200
1	14	5	25–100
2	10	4	25–200
1	27	2.5	35–100
3	10	2	35–100
4	7	4	15–100
1	13	6	35–200
3	10	2	35–100
0	16	7	25–50

On the other hand, if you're looking for a meal replacement, high-protein bars can pack as much power as that tuna sandwich you meant to eat for lunch. The Daily Value (DV) for protein is 50 grams, but as a fitness enthusiast, you need 75 to 100 grams daily. Some bars supply close to half that.

In addition, check the ingredients list for the source of protein. Most bars use a lactose-free milk protein, which is a good source of essential amino acids. Soy, another protein source that provides extra disease-fighting powers, is found in bars such as GeniSoy and PR Bar. Studies show that isoflavones in soy may reduce your risk for certain types of cancer. They also may lower blood cholesterol levels and heart disease risk and slow the progression of osteoporosis.

Carbohydrate. Energy bars contain 20 to 50 grams of carbohydrate. When you work out for extended periods of time, your body needs 30 to 60 grams per hour of exercise. You'll stay well-fueled by eating an energy bar per hour while running or doing other intense workouts.

Most bars combine complex carbohydrate like those in rice, oats, or other starchy foods with the simple carbohydrate found in dried fruit, brown-rice syrup, or high-fructose corn syrup. If you prefer natural ingredients, stick with bars such as Clif and Stoker that contain no high-fructose corn sweetener or refined ingredients.

Fiber. Too much fiber may slow your digestion, keeping fuel from getting to your muscles as fast as you need it. It also can make you take extra pit stops during a race or workout. So choose bars with 5 grams of fiber or less to eat during your workout. When eating an energy bar as a snack or in place of a meal, however, select one with more fiber. It'll make you feel full longer.

Fat. Look for bars with 4 grams of fat or less for every 230 calories. Fat slows digestion, which keeps fuel from getting to your muscles as quickly as you need it. (It also can make you feel nauseated during a workout.) If you are watching your blood cholesterol levels, be aware that a handful of brands contain artery-clogging saturated fat.

Manufacturers of bars with a 40-30-30 distribution of calories from carbohydrate, protein, and fat claim that these bars (in tandem with a 40-30-30 diet plan) assist in burning body fat. So far, however, research has not supported these claims.

Fortification. Some energy bars are crammed with as many vitamins and minerals as a bowl of fortified breakfast cereal or even a multivitamin. Extra antioxidants, including vitamins C, E, and beta-carotene, help your body recover from exercise. If you are using an energy bar as a snack or to replace a meal, this vitamin and mineral fortification can help make up for what you are not getting through food.

Beyond vitamins and minerals, some manufacturers add extras such as ginseng or other herbs, amino acids, and specialty ingredients not found in the traditional energy bar. For the most part, the amounts of these ingredients are too small to provide a benefit.

Making the Best of Bars

Energy bars are a convenient addition to your diet as a healthful snack. Use these tips when choosing a bar to fit your needs.

- Drink 12 to 16 ounces of water with an energy bar, whether you're eating it while working out or while sitting at your desk.
- During exercise, take one bite at a time and rewrap your bar if you find it difficult to chomp down all at once. Your goal is to eat one bar during every hour of exercise, not one bar in 5 minutes.
- Throw out your energy bar if you've taken a bite out of it and let it sit for a few hours. This will help you avoid any bacteria that may have started to grow. When unopened, however, an energy bar is an ideal "traveling" fuel that doesn't require refrigeration.
- Get back in touch with fruits, vegetables, and other whole foods when the energy bar wrappers in your garbage can, on your car floor, or in your gym bag outnumber the remnants of real food.

Sports Drinks

Serving size: 8 ounces **Calories:** 50 to 80 **Carbohydrate:** 12 to 19 grams
Extras: Sodium, potassium, vitamins

In workouts lasting an hour or more, you need to replenish carbohydrate as well as water. Sports drinks provide both. Does this mean that sports drinks allow you to exercise longer? In a word, yes.

In one study, researchers at Georgia State University in Atlanta asked men and women to run on a treadmill for 90 minutes at about 70 percent of their maximum effort. Then they ran a 10-K time trial. During the entire session, runners drank either a sports drink or a placebo beverage, consuming about 6 ounces of fluid every 15 minutes.

The sports drink group ran the 10-K significantly faster than the placebo group. Moreover, those who downed the sports drink rated their efforts as being easier than the placebo group did. And despite the large volume of ingested fluid, the runners had no stomach discomfort.

When considering what sports drink might be best for you, follow these tips.

Check the percentage of carbohydrate. During exercise, you want a drink with 5 to 8 percent carbohydrate. Anything above 8 percent slows digestion and promotes cramping, nausea, and diarrhea. Anything below 5 per-

Sports Drink Rundown

If you don't want to examine the labels on every single sports drink at the store—and there are plenty—relax. I've done it for you. Here is the calorie and carbohydrate content in 11 popular drinks. All figures are for an 8-ounce serving.

Drink	Calories	Carbohydrate (g)
Allsport	70	19
Cytomax	80	19
Endura	62	16
Gatorade	50	14
Hydra Fuel	70	17
Isostar	70	16
Met-Rx ORS	75	19
Perform	60	16
Powerade	70	19
PowerSurge	80	20
Race Day	63	15

cent won't get enough fuel to your muscles. To figure out the percentage of carbohydrate in a drink, divide the grams of carbohydrate per serving by the milliliters of drink per serving and multiply by 100. For example, if a sports drink has 14 grams of carbohydrate per 240 milliliter serving, divide 14 by 240. Then multiply that answer (.058) by 100. You end up with 5.8, which means that the drink is nearly 6 percent carbohydrate.

Before and after exercise, your body can handle more carbohydrate. Drinks such as Iorq, Gatorload, and HydraFuel are designed specifically for this purpose. Many people have trouble stomaching solid food just before or after exercise, especially on a hot day. These high-carbohydrate drinks, with 40 to 60 grams per 8 ounces, provide the perfect solution. Just don't drink them *during* exercise; they'll sit in your stomach.

Look for sodium. Many sports drinks contain sodium, potassium, and other electrolytes that help promote body fluid balance. You don't need a lot, but a small amount of sodium serves three important functions: It makes you thirsty, which encourages you to drink more; it retains water, preventing dehydration and annoying pit stops; and it replaces some of the sodium you lose through sweat. Look for a drink with 100 to 110 milligrams of sodium per 8-ounce serving. If you're worried about increasing your risk of high blood pressure, that's the same amount of sodium as in 8 ounces of 2% milk, and is only $\frac{1}{10}$ of your daily requirement. You also want other electrolytes, such as potassium and chloride, in the drink. Look for a drink that includes about 30 milligrams of potassium per 8-ounce serving.

Check the type of carbohydrate. Some research shows that your digestive tract does better with a blend of different kinds of carbohydrate than it does with just one type. Check the ingredients list for different sugars such as sucrose, fructose, glucose, and maltodextrin. Avoid drinks with a high concentration of fructose (a fruit sugar), which can slow hydration and contribute to intestinal trouble. If combined with other sugars, however, fructose rarely causes discomfort. Just make sure it's not the first or only sugar listed.

Avoid carbonation. The bubbles in carbonated drinks can make you feel gassy and even nauseated. They can also discourage you from drinking because carbonated beverages are not easy to chug.

workout q&a

Q: Aren't drinks that contain fruit sugar (fructose) more nutritious than those that contain table sugar? Wouldn't I be better off simply diluting some apple or cranberry juice?

A: No. The best type of carbohydrate for exercise is the kind that is easily broken down and absorbed by your intestines. The sugar found in fruit, called fructose, actually slows down water and energy absorption, hampering energy and fluid delivery to your muscles. Research shows that a drink made exclusively with fructose may actually upset your stomach.

A small amount of fructose in a sports drink won't cause problems as long as there are other, more easily absorbed sugars also present. Most sports drinks are made with sucrose (table sugar), glucose (the sugar used by your body as fuel), and some fructose. Maltodextrin, also called glucose polymers, is added to some sports drinks. Simply check the label to be sure that fructose is not the first ingredient listed.

Buy what tastes best. Studies show that you'll drink more if you like the taste of the drink. Experiment with different flavors and brands; try them when sitting around the house and while exercising. Studies show that people rate the taste of a drink differently depending on whether they are drinking during a workout or after one.

Drink the right amount. Sports drinks will provide the most benefit during workouts that last longer than an hour. You should consume 5 to 12 ounces of a sports drink every 15 minutes.

Fitness Water

Serving size: 8 ounces   **Calories:** 10   **Carbohydrate:** 2 grams
Extras: Sodium, potassium, B vitamins, vitamins C and E

Until recently, people who exercised for an hour or less were stranded in the land of hydration boredom. They didn't need the calories of a sports drink, yet didn't want to drink tasteless water. So, many of them, despite good intentions, lived in a chronically dehydrated state.

Now, there is another option: fitness water. Propel Fitness Water, from the makers of Gatorade, is available in berry, orange, and lime flavors, and contains only 10 calories per 8 ounces. It also has a dash of sodium and potassium, a handful of B vitamins, and the antioxidants C and E.

If you're a fitness enthusiast who's out there for less than an hour, fitness water is perfect for you. The electrolytes will help you retain more fluid, and the flavor encourages you to drink more. It also makes a great low-calorie beverage to sip throughout the day.

Energy Gels

Serving size: One packet   **Calories:** 80 to 133   **Carbohydrate:** 20 to 28 grams
Extras: Caffeine, branched-chain amino acids, antioxidants, herbs, lactic acid "buffering" agents

Energy gels are a relatively new concept in body fueling. Puddinglike in texture, gels are fairly easy to eat and digest, and they're simple to transport. Gels typically weigh about 1 ounce per packet, so you can easily tuck a few into the waistband of your shorts for quick refueling. Just remember that you still need to drink water, since gels by themselves won't keep you hydrated.

Each packet of gel contains 80 to 133 calories and 20 to 28 grams of carbohydrate per serving. Consisting partly of simple sugars, gels are absorbed directly into the bloodstream and provide instant energy. With the addition of electrolytes (such as potassium) in most gels and caffeine in some, they provide a total performance package.

And they work. In one study, runners took either an energy gel and water or an artificially sweetened placebo drink during a 2-hour treadmill run. The gel users downed one packet (100 calories from 25 grams of carbohydrate) every 30 minutes, along with an adequate amount of water. Compared to the placebo group, the gel users maintained higher blood sugar levels, which suggests that the gel had been digested and was available to the muscles as an energy source. The researchers didn't assess performance, but it is likely that the gel would have helped because of its effect on blood glucose.

If the price of gels—$1 or more per pack—keeps you from using these refueling gems, try honey, a natural energy gel. Available in packets or sticks that contain about 1 teaspoon and 25 calories, you'll need two per half-hour.

But why fuel up on gels instead of energy bars when you head into your second hour of exercise? Both forms of carbohydrate are good sources of energy, but sucking down a gel is easier for many people than gnawing on a bar. Furthermore, the fiber, protein, and fat in bars can sometimes slow the absorption process, resulting in a slower release of energy. Sports drinks work well, too, but they are tough to carry during some types of exercise.

During exercise, you need to consume 30 to 60 grams of carbohydrate per hour to keep your body running and your energy high. That amounts to one or two gels an hour. Because gels have such a strong concentration of carbohydrate, swallow them along with 8 ounces of water to help them move through your stomach and into your intestines quickly—plan to pop a pouch just before hitting a water fountain.

And experiment. Test out different brands and different flavors to see what you like best. The tastes and textures of gels vary widely, from chocolate to pineapple, and from pudding to liquid. Let your palate be the judge. Packaging also varies; some gels are easier to open than others. You'll be ingesting the gels while moving, so the ease with which you can rip open the pouch and squeeze out the gel (without dribbling half of it down your chin) is key. Here's more of what to look for when choosing gels.

Caffeine. Research has long shown that drinking a cup or two of coffee just before exercise encourages the release of fatty acids into your blood. Your muscles then use these fatty acids for fuel, which conserves glycogen, your muscles' regular fuel source. In practical terms, you can work out longer without feeling tired.

But no research has studied whether the ingestion of caffeine during exercise triggers the same effect. The gels that contain caffeine include only 25 milligrams per packet, the amount in a ¼ cup of coffee. That's probably not enough to boost your endurance.

It may be enough to cause some other problems, however. Many

A New Twist on an Old Favorite

Most folks are familiar with ice pops made out of fruit juice. But how about a frozen pop made with your favorite sports drink? Pour about 4 ounces of sports drink into a paper cup and put it in your freezer. After about 45 minutes, when the liquid has become slushy, place a Popsicle stick in the center and continue freezing. Then, after a workout—or anytime—peel away the paper and enjoy.

people have complained of a laxative effect when they take these gels. My suggestion: If you want to give caffeinated gels a try, consume them during a low-key exercise session where you have easy access to a bathroom.

Branched-chain amino acids. Two of the most popular sports gels on the market—Gu and PowerGel—both contain these building blocks of protein. Some experts theorize that your body will burn these amino acids (leucine, valine, and isoleucine) once it runs out of stored carbohydrate. And some studies do show that the ingestion of branched-chain amino acids during exercise can delay fatigue (other studies have shown the opposite). Because there's no evidence that branched-chain amino acids hurt your performance, there's no reason to avoid them; realistically, they are present in such small amounts that they are unlikely to do any harm or good.

Antioxidants and herbs. Some companies add vitamins C and E to their gels to reduce the oxidative damage of exercise, although whether it helps to take these vitamins during your workout is still up in the air. But because most people don't get enough vitamin E in their regular diets, if a gel contains this important heart disease fighter, I'm all for it.

Acid buffers. When you exercise, your muscle fluids and blood become slightly acidic from the buildup of lactic acid. This is why you "feel the burn" during long or intense workouts. Some energy gels contain ingredients that help neutralize your blood acidity, although it's not known for sure whether these buffering agents boost your performance or just delay fatigue.

chapter ten

The Science of Supplements

I t'll make you fast, lean, and strong. Do you want some? Who wouldn't? That kind of marketing is hard to resist—an estimated 40 percent or more of people living in the United States take some form of dietary supplement. The problem is that with more than 29,000 supplements to choose from, separating what you need from what the manufacturers want you to *think* you need can be tricky.

Sorting through the Hype

Unlike the restrictions put on food products, the FDA allows supplement manufacturers to make virtually any claim other than that their product can prevent a disease. These structure-and-function claims, as they're called, generally suggest that a supplement improves the body's functioning. For example, a supplement might say that it boosts immune health rather than state that it prevents bacterial infection.

The FDA doesn't regulate supplements because they fall into an odd category. They are definitely not a food, but because they are available over the counter, they are not classified as drugs. The FDA does evaluate structure-and-function claims and will pursue a supplement company over consumer complaints or if adverse side effects occur. From time to time, the FDA will issue statements regarding specific supplements, especially if it considers them dangerous. Still, as a smart consumer, you should keep in mind that when a supplement claim sounds too good to be true, it usually is. Be on the lookout for words and phrases such as "breakthrough," "magical," "miracle cure," and "new discovery."

In addition, testing has shown that many supplements don't contain the active ingredients that are listed on the labels. (To see how various brands stack up, go to www.consumerlab.com.) Many supplements claim to do amazing things for your body with virtually no science to back them up, so you'll need to do your own research to make sure you get what you pay for.

Who Needs Them?

Most people who supplement don't need to, and most who don't supplement should, says hematologist Randy Eichner, M.D., at the University of Oklahoma Medical Center in Oklahoma City. Besides getting a blood test, how can you find out if you are deficient in a particular nutrient? Some things make it more likely.

1. Dieting. If you restrict your daily caloric intake to fewer than 1,200, you're likely missing out on several important nutrients.
2. Lactose intolerance. If you can't eat dairy products, you may fall short on calcium and riboflavin.
3. Food allergies. If you can't eat particular foods such as wheat and fruit, you'll have a tougher time getting some of the nutrients you need.
4. Vegetarian diet. Going without meat makes it harder to get enough iron and zinc, especially if you're female. You also may come up short on vitamins B_{12} (not found in plant foods) and D as well as riboflavin.
5. Pregnancy. Supplement with iron and folic acid or eat fortified cereals just in case, and follow your physician's advice on prenatal supplements.

In addition, some supplements may offer therapeutic benefits that you can't get from food alone. For example, you won't find glucosamine in any food. But the supplement may do wonders for your joint health without the side effects of common prescription medications.

23 Popular Supplements

The claims made for some supplements are seriously far-fetched, but a handful of others have grabbed the attention of scientists as well as athletes because studies have shown promising results. To set the record straight, here's a close look at 23 of the most popular supplements on the shelves. If you have any doubts about whether a particular supplement is right for you, ask your physician.

Androstenedione

Better known as andro, this supplement made headlines when baseball slugger Mark McGwire said that andro, along with the supplement creatine, helped him to build muscle mass. Andro quickly sold out of stores while scientists tried to find out whether the supplement worked and if it was safe.

In both cases, the verdict was no. Natural androstenedione is a hormone secreted by your adrenal glands. Companies who make the supplement claim that supplemental andro boosts levels of the hormone testosterone, helping to build muscle mass and sex drive. But when scientists tested it in the lab, they found that the supplement did not improve muscle mass, body composition, or libido. It did lower healthy HDL cholesterol levels, however.

One study published in the prestigious *Journal of the American Medical Association* found that while andro did not boost testosterone or muscle mass, it did boost estrogen, which is dangerous for men. Among other things, the supplement may increase the risk of male breast enlargement, cancer, and heart disease.

My recommendation: Leave andro to gather dust on the restocked shelves.

Branched-Chain Amino Acids

Branched-chain amino acids, or BCAAs, have been a hot topic for years, and they do show promise for endurance athletes. Several well-designed studies suggest that supplemental BCAAs may improve your exercise performance and help prevent the muscle damage that can occur with heavy training.

BCAAs, along with 17 other amino acids, are the building blocks that form all of the protein in your body. They come mostly from meats and beans; and during 2 or more hours of exercise, your body breaks down these amino acids and burns them for energy. If this happens often enough, your muscle protein supply starts to dwindle. Taking a BCAA supplement might help.

Researchers from the University of Tasmania in Australia investigated the effects of BCAA supplementation on muscle damage in a group of cyclists. The cyclists took either a placebo or 12 grams (double the amount from dietary sources) of BCAAs daily for 6 days. Immediately following the supplementation period, they cycled hard for 2 hours. After this exercise session, researchers took blood samples every hour for several hours, then once a day for 4 days. The researchers then measured muscle-tissue damage based on various enzyme levels in the blood. Compared to the placebo group, cyclists who took BCAA supplements showed less muscle damage, leading researchers to believe that the supplement may have helped replace the BCAAs lost during exercise.

Before you try BCAA supplementation, remember that by far the best way to maintain adequate muscle tissue is by getting enough calories and protein. And while those in the study had no adverse side effects from BCAA supplementation, 6 days is hardly enough time to determine long-term side effects.

My recommendation: Although branched-chain amino acids show promise, especially for endurance athletes, wait for more research to determine the safety of this supplement before you start popping one every day. Instead, make sure you are eating 75 to 100 grams of protein a day.

Calcium

Calcium always has been and always will be the mineral for bone health. And bone health is not just a woman's issue. Sure, osteoporosis is a bigger concern for women, but both male and female bones lose calcium as they age.

workout q&a

Q: • My breakfast cereal and energy bars are fortified with vitamins and minerals.
• I also take a daily multivitamin and drink a nutrient-rich fruit smoothie every day. Is it possible to suffer a vitamin overdose from all of these fortified foods?

A: Yes, it is. For many nutrients, more does not mean better. In fact, consuming some vitamins and minerals in amounts beyond the Daily Value (DV) could lead to toxicity. Vitamins A and D, for example, in amounts as low as three times the DV, can be dangerous, especially to children. Also, just two servings of fortified breakfast cereal dumps enough iron in your system to block the absorption of the mineral zinc, which is crucial for a strong immune system.

Besides a possible vitamin and mineral overdose, reaching for an antioxidant-fortified food bar instead of a naturally antioxidant-packed orange or carrot may shortchange your health. According to researchers, it may be the unique interaction of these antioxidants and other nutrients found in perfect balance only in produce and a few other real foods that helps reduce cancer and heart disease risk. Once you take these nutrients out of their natural form and process them into a pill, shake, or bar, they may lose some of their healing properties.

To make sure fortified foods don't overtake your diet, follow these tips.

- Reach for real food first. Eat a minimum of five fruit and vegetable servings and at least eight servings of whole grains daily.
- Vary your selections of cereals, fortified beverages, and other vitamin-boosted foods and feel free to go for nonfortified foods as well.
- Skip your daily multivitamin/mineral supplement if you eat fortified breakfast cereal or other vitamin-enhanced food.

As a fitness enthusiast, you should be especially concerned about your bones. Any weight-bearing, repetitive exercise can strengthen your bones, but an overuse injury such as a shinsplint can turn into a stress fracture, especially if you're not eating enough calcium.

Besides protecting your bones, calcium also regulates blood pressure, prevents colon cancer, and may even aid weight loss, so get plenty of calcium. Make dairy products such as low-fat milk, yogurt, cheese, and cottage cheese a part of your daily menu. Even if you have a lactose intolerance, you may be able to consume 8 ounces or more of milk or yogurt a day without symptoms if you spread out your intake. You can use lactose-free milk or Lactaid-type products. Also look for calcium-fortified soy milk and orange juice, plus tofu, canned salmon, broccoli, and tortillas made with lime.

My recommendation: Aim for 1,000 to 1,500 milligrams a day. That amounts to three to five glasses of milk a day. If you don't think you're getting that much from food, consider a 500-milligram supplement. Taking the supplement with dinner will ensure the best absorption because for most people, dinner is the meal with the lowest calcium content.

Carbohydrate

While they may not be found in the supplement aisle of your local supermarket or health food store, some sports products have introduced the idea of carbo-loading as a form of supplementation. If your body is not well-stocked with carbohydrate, you're not going to exercise well. You need plenty of carbohydrate to replenish the glycogen stores in your muscles to fuel your workout, or your arms and legs will feel heavy and you won't feel like working out for very long. But do you need to take a carbohydrate supplement such as the drink Gatorload? It depends.

Aim for 400 carbohydrate grams (1,600 calories) as a daily goal—more if you do high mileage or if you eat considerably more than 2,500 total calories a day. To figure out your daily average, keep track of your carbohydrate servings for 2 or 3 days in a row. You'll know you're on the right track if you come close to the following numbers each day.

- 10 servings of grains (one slice of bread or ½ cup of cereal or pasta equals 1 serving)
- 7 servings of fruit (one medium-size piece or 4 ounces of juice equals 1 serving)
- 4 servings of vegetables (1 cup raw or ½ cup cooked equals 1 serving)
- 2 to 3 servings of dairy (1 cup equals 1 serving)

My recommendation: If you don't come close to the recommended amount of carbohydrate and you exercise for an hour or more at a time, consider drinking a carbohydrate-loaded beverage such as Gatorload before or after your workouts.

Chromium

Chromium has been around the research block a few times. For years, the mineral was rumored to help burn body fat and build muscle size and strength, which appealed to those looking for a stronger, shapelier body. But before you sprint to the nearest nutrition depot, here's a look at the facts.

Chromium assists the hormone insulin in processing carbohydrates. Insulin also helps your body manufacture new proteins, a fact that supports the theory of chromium as a muscle builder.

Unfortunately, that theory just doesn't pan out. Much of the initial chromium craze was based on a slew of flawed studies showing that chromium supplementation (in the form of chromium picolinate) improved muscle gains during strength training. Yet in a well-designed study on football players, those who weight trained 4 days a week while taking 200 micrograms of chromium saw no increase in their muscle mass compared to a placebo group. But while most research has failed to support chromium for fat burning or muscle building, the supplement may show promise in another area: Research suggests that this supplement might be useful for boosting sprint performance.

Chromium is a trace mineral that helps your cells use carbohydrate for energy. Along with the hormone insulin, chromium acts like a key that unlocks cells, allowing sugar to enter. This explains why blood sugar levels improve in people with diabetes who are given extra chromium in their diets. Using this logic, it makes sense that an extra shot of chromium during exercise could help shuttle more carbohydrate into muscle cells for a boost of energy.

Researchers from the University of Dayton in Ohio put this theory to the test with a group of trained cyclists. On two separate occasions, cyclists worked out for an hour while they drank either a high-carbohydrate beverage similar to a sports drink or the same beverage with added

chromium. They consumed about 60 grams of carbohydrate (240 calories) and about 200 micrograms of chromium (equivalent to the daily recommended intake).

At the end of the hour-long ride, cyclists pedaled as hard as they
could for just under a minute. Researchers measured the amount of work
performed during the sprint and found that the chromium-fortified drink
boosted sprint performance by 7 percent over the plain carbohydrate
drink. Blood sugar levels were also slightly lower in the cyclists who had
used the chromium-fortified beverage, suggesting that more glucose had
been used by the muscles. Lead researcher Mary Ellen Horn, R.D., notes,
"Under these conditions, it appears that a modest chromium dose improves glucose uptake for use during a sprint effort."

My recommendation: You don't need to buy a supplement to increase your daily chromium intake; you get 50 to 60 micrograms of
chromium from 1 cup of refried beans, two microbrewed beers, a cooked
chicken breast, or 1 cup of peas.

To keep your chromium levels optimal (many endurance athletes do
fall short of the recommended 50 to 200 micrograms), beware of eating
too many refined foods, such as white bread and sweets, which are not
only low in chromium but also may boost your need for it (to help
process carbohydrates). Sticking with food sources instead of a supplement is both cheaper and safer. If you consume too much chromium
(which can happen only if you supplement), you can hamper your absorption of iron and zinc.

Creatine

Creatine may be one of the best-selling supplements ever, with more
than $100 million in annual sales. Athletes everywhere are using it, with
good reason. According to manufacturers' labels, loading up on creatine
for several days boosts muscle strength and sprint performance. When
taken for a few weeks, creatine may even pump up muscle size.

All of this hype is real. Many studies suggest quite strongly that creatine works. The only catch is that it might not work for everyone.

Manufactured by your body, creatine is a proteinlike substance also
found in fish, beef, and other meats. In your muscles, creatine acts much

like the cylinders in your car's engine, helping fire up your muscles during high-intensity exercise such as weight lifting, jumping, or sprinting. Load up with creatine from a supplement (20 to 25 grams daily for 5 to 7 days), and you boost the number of cylinders in your muscles.

After the loading phase, a maintenance dose of 2 to 5 grams a day helps maintain those high levels, resulting in more strength and a greater ability to do single or repeated bouts of high-effort exercise such as sprinting. As an added benefit, creatine supplements taken over several weeks may boost levels of HDL (good) cholesterol. And since men typically have lower HDL levels than women, this possible benefit of creatine increases its appeal to male athletes.

It sounds alluring, but it doesn't work for everyone. Endurance athletes are the clear losers in the creatine story. For starters, creatine loading may make you gain weight, which can make you feel sluggish. In fact, creatine loading in swimmers does not appear to consistently boost sprint performance, and it may even have a negative impact because weight gain can change body position in the water.

Research shows only that loading up on creatine helps during weight lifting and during brief, high-intensity exercise typically lasting less than a minute. Dosing with creatine has not been shown to have any performance-enhancing powers for longer efforts, especially continuous exercise such as long-distance running and cycling.

My recommendation: Give creatine a try if you're interested in increasing the size of your muscles or if you want to run sprints. But if you're keeping your weight down for the next marathon, stick with a high-carbohydrate diet.

Fat Blockers

Made from chitosan, a type of fiber from shrimp and crab shells, these supplements claim to stop your intestines from absorbing fat, which should lower the number of calories that enter your body. The theory is that chitosan's large, bulky chemical structure acts much like a sticky piece of Velcro that traps small amounts of fatty substances in your intestines. The chitosan, along with the fat and cholesterol, doesn't get absorbed by your intestines; instead, it all ends up in your stool. As a result, calories get sucked out of your body before they can be absorbed.

That all sounds great until you stop and think about it. If weight loss were really that easy, everyone would be as skinny as a supermodel. The fact is that it's not that easy.

Over several weeks, researchers fed laboratory mice a high-fat diet that was 10 to 15 percent chitosan by weight. The animals gained significantly less fat than control mice eating the same fat-laden diet. This may sound promising, but the mice ate large amounts of chitosan (much more than the recommended amount on many product labels), which resulted in large amounts of fat being excreted in their feces. In humans, this condition of excessive fat in the stool is called steatorrhea, which is not only uncomfortable but also embarrassing.

Studies done on people are few and far between, and the results are less promising than those done on mice. One study concluded that chitosan doesn't work for people, period. Other research shows that chitosan may be able to bind 3 to 4 grams of fat per meal at most. That amounts to a mere 30 calories—half the amount in a banana. That's hardly a situation where you can eat anything you want and still lose weight.

Chitosan may be more promising for your heart health, however. While the men in one study didn't lose weight, their blood cholesterol levels fell significantly. Levels of the good HDL cholesterol rose, which suggests that chitosan may have the potential to lower cholesterol. But it may also lower your absorption of fat-soluble vitamins (such as vitamin E) and cause intestinal yeast overgrowth.

My Food Diary

I'm not a pill popper, and never have been. In fact, I even find it hard to stay on any type of prescription medication. I've tried off and on to take daily doses of glucosamine and chondroitin sulfate, but I always seem to fall off the supplement wagon.

While my eating habits are usually healthful at home, they go down the drain when I'm on the road. Because I may be guest-hosting a radio show as late as midnight or 2:00 A.M., my eating is sporadic, so I take a multivitamin/mineral supplement when I travel. I also take 400 IU of vitamin E every 3 to 4 days to replace what I would otherwise have gotten from whole grains and nuts.

Besides chitosan, there are many brands of fat blockers on the market. The packaging for these generally proclaim that the products "block fat absorption."

My recommendation: Fat-blocker pills cost about $10 for a 1-week supply, so spend your money on something more worthwhile.

Fat Burners

Log on to the Internet, flip through a fitness magazine, or cruise the supplement aisles in a health food store, and you're bound to come across a staggering array of supplements that claim to speed your metabolism and shed unwanted fat.

Many of these products contain a Chinese herb called ma huang, also called ephedra, or a synthetic version called ephedrine. Caffeine is a common ingredient as well. These ingredients show promise as weight-loss aids, but they also have been proven to be dangerous—and even deadly—for some users.

Both ephedrine and caffeine are powerful central nervous system stimulants, which means that they increase heart rate and blood pressure as well as boost your calorie burn. How they do this isn't clear, but research indicates that they introduce an inefficiency to the body so that it wastes heat energy.

A handful of studies show that weight-loss claims are valid when these supplements are combined with a low-calorie diet. When combined with caffeine, ephedra does enhance fat loss, suppress appetite, and stimulate fat burning beyond what would normally happen on a restricted-calorie diet. In one study, people lost 36 pounds during the 6 months that they took a daily caffeine-and-ephedrine supplement; the placebo group lost 29 pounds.

The problem with this is that the dose that produces this effect is 60 milligrams of ephedrine and 600 milligrams of caffeine, which is the amount in 6 cups of coffee. Many people who take ephedrine and caffeine report that both can cause a speeding heart rate, dizziness, sweating, and other symptoms of nervousness. The FDA has been notified of more than 800 adverse side effects, including heart attack, stroke, tremors, and insomnia. A total of 17 deaths have been blamed on the use of ephedrine, either as an ingredient in a supplement or as a supplement itself.

The FDA recommends that consumers avoid all types of ephedra products, including many weight-loss formulas, and it will soon limit supplements to 8 milligrams of ephedrine per serving and a maximum daily dose of 24 milligrams.

My recommendation: Stay away from these products.

Fish Oil

A type of oil called omega-3 fatty acid, which is found in fish such as salmon and tuna, can lower your blood cholesterol. As a fitness enthusiast, you should be interested in fish oil for a different reason: its anti-inflammatory action. An omega-3 fatty acid supplement of 1 to 1½ grams a day may reduce joint pain and rheumatoid arthritis symptoms, and even help those with psoriasis and inflammatory bowel disorders. Think of it as a natural painkiller for your sore, overworked muscles.

Fish oil may work by affecting the prostaglandin levels in your body. Different types of prostaglandins signal different bodily responses. Some tell your tissues to swell up; others tell those same tissues to calm down. Researchers suspect that years of eating too much of omega-6 fatty acids (found in vegetable oils) and too little of omega-3's may bring on inflammation.

Omega-6 fats are not bad fats; they can be quite healthy. Most of us are out of balance, however. Scientists suspect that the healthiest ratio of these fats is four omega-6's to every one omega-3. That doesn't sound hard to follow until you learn that the typical diet in the United States contains about 10 omega-6's to one omega-3.

My recommendation: Don't run out to the store, buy a bottle of fish oil supplements, and down the whole thing at once. For fish oil to work, you need to increase omega-3's while decreasing the saturated fats found in butter, the trans fats found in processed foods, and the omega-6 fatty acids found in vegetable oil. So as you supplement with up to 2 grams a day of omega-3's, cut back on other, less healthful fats. And bump up your intake of fish and flaxseed meal or oil to two servings a week.

Taking lots of fish oil supplements can have not-so-nice side effects such as bad breath, body odor, and diarrhea. Look for enteric-coated, delayed release capsules, which will help offset those side effects, and make an effort to eat real fish rather than relying on supplements.

Folate (Folic Acid)

Researchers have been touting the importance of this B vitamin for years, and with good reason. Women who don't get enough folate before and during pregnancy increase their risk of having babies with birth defects, and both men and women who skimp on folate increase their risk of heart disease. Among women and men, folate keeps blood cells healthy and fights off a severe form of anemia, which can make you drag through your workouts.

My recommendation: While folate is relatively scarce in foods, the FDA's folate-fortification program requires all enriched grain products (bread, cereal, pasta) to be fortified with folate. Including any of those products daily will help you meet the Daily Value (DV) of 400 micrograms. Other good folate sources include green, leafy vegetables; lentils; fortified cereals; and citrus fruits.

Ginseng

You can find ginseng everywhere: in sports drinks, iced tea, herbal supplements, and energy gels. Used for thousands of years in China, ginseng is an herb traditionally taken to remedy chronic fatigue, nervous disorders, low sex drive, and forgetfulness. In terms of exercise, ginseng has been said to boost energy levels and performance and to speed workout recovery. But aside from anecdotes and testimonials, there is no evidence that supports ginseng's performance-boosting effects.

Research has been done, however. H. J. Engels, Ph.D., an exercise physiologist at Wayne State University in Detroit, tested ginseng on a group of female athletes. Each athlete took either 200 milligrams of ginseng extract or a placebo daily for 8 weeks. The women then pedaled to exhaustion on stationary bikes while being monitored for performance factors during and immediately after exercise. The ginseng provided no performance or recovery benefit.

In another study, Dr. Engels looked at whether ginseng improves mood and whether it has a positive effect on perceived exertion. Again, researchers used an 8-week supplementation period and the same bike test. The results of this study showed that the herb provided no lift in mood, nor did the subjects feel that they were pedaling more easily.

On the other hand, ginseng might help you somewhat if you play a sport that requires a lot of hand-eye coordination. In one small study, researchers tested the reaction time of soccer players who had supplemented with either 350 milligrams of ginseng or a placebo for 6 weeks. They asked the soccer players to ride stationary bikes. During the strenuous workout, the soccer players who had taken the ginseng had faster reaction times than those who had taken the placebo.

My recommendation: Save your money for something more worthwhile. Ginseng has a long history as a medicinal herb, but it hasn't been scientifically shown to provide any performance benefit.

Glucosamine and Chondroitin Sulfate

Glucosamine is an amino acid sugar that acts as the structural component of tendons, ligaments, and cartilage. Chondroitin is a component of cartilage. According to the manufacturers' claims, when taken together, these two supplements protect joints and tendons and relieve osteoarthritis pain.

In the past few years, orthopedists and other physicians have increasingly advised patients to take both glucosamine and chondroitin sulfate to ease the inflammation and pain of osteoarthritis, a degenerative joint condition caused by overuse, traumatic injury, or old age. One of the hallmarks of osteoarthritis is an erosion of the cartilage that cushions your joints. Chondrocytes—the cells in your joints that make cartilage—need glucosamine to function optimally. According to several studies, about 1,500 milligrams each of supplemental glucosamine and chondroitin daily helps soothe pain, possibly by stimulating cartilage growth. Animal studies also suggest that supplemental glucosamine may speed the repair of injured joints.

Glucosamine also helps produce substances in ligaments, tendons, and joint fluids called glycoproteins, so it may speed healing in those areas as well. Research has yet to test that theory, however.

Recipe Revver

Powerhouse Salad
Serves 4

This salad contains more vitamins, minerals, and antioxidants than most supplements you can buy at the store. In particular, it's loaded with vitamins A, B$_6$, E, and K along with folate and fiber. I recommend eating it on a regular basis.

Dressing

- 3 tablespoons rice wine vinegar
- 1 tablespoon balsamic vinegar
- 1 teaspoon sesame oil
- 2 teaspoons canola oil
  Salt and pepper (optional)

Salad

- ⅔ cup shelled, whole soybeans
- 8 cups spring mix (arugula, spinach, kale, romaine, endive, radicchio)
- 1 red tomato, chopped into bite-size pieces
- 1 yellow tomato, chopped into bite-size pieces
- 1 red bell pepper, seeded and chopped
- ½ cup grated carrots
- ⅓ cup chopped broccoli
- 2 ounces goat cheese, crumbled
- 2 ounces roasted, chopped almonds

To make the dressing: In a small jar with a lid, combine the rice wine vinegar, balsamic vinegar, sesame oil, canola oil, and salt and pepper (if using), and shake well.

To make the salad: Cook the soybeans according to the package directions and allow to cool. In a large salad bowl, combine the soybeans, spring mix, red and yellow tomatoes, pepper, carrots, and broccoli. Pour the dressing over the salad and toss well. Sprinkle the goat cheese and almonds on top. Serve immediately.

Per serving: *280 calories, 14 g protein, 19 g carbohydrate, 17 g total fat, 4 g saturated fat, 11 mg cholesterol, 7 g dietary fiber, 114 mg sodium*

My recommendation: Consult your physician if you want to give glucosamine and chondroitin sulfate a try. Few studies have looked at the safety of this supplement. In one small study, a group of people with diabetes who took glucosamine experienced lower insulin sensitivity and blood sugar control, so if you have diabetes, I strongly urge you to talk with your doctor before taking this supplement. These pills come with a hefty price tag, and you may have to take them three times a day. If you decide to take glucosamine and chondroitin supplements, take 1,200 to 1,500 milligrams of each per day.

Glutamine

Found abundantly in your muscles and blood plasma, the nonessential amino acid glutamine serves as fuel for your immune cells. Because physical stress and heavy exercise deplete glutamine from your plasma, some researchers suspect that supplementing with this amino acid may ward off colds and muscle soreness induced by endurance exercise.

While few studies have been done on this supplement, research does suggest that supplemental glutamine improves your immune function and response to infections. A study published in *The Journal of Applied Physiology* found that the addition of glutamine to a carbohydrate beverage (such as a sports drink) could help you recover faster. Another study, published in the journal *Nutrition*, found that a total of 10 milligrams of the supplement taken after exhaustive exercise such as a marathon could cut the risk of catching a cold in half.

My recommendation: Take 5 to 20 grams after endurance exercise such as a 4-hour bike ride or 2-hour run. This supplement is no substitute for rest and a proper recovery diet, however.

Iron

You must have an adequate amount of iron in your blood to get oxygen to your muscles. If you don't get enough, you experience extreme fatigue, lagging performances, and are often more susceptible to colds. Since you may be losing some iron in your sweat and urine, and because exercise itself can hamper your ability to absorb the mineral, you need to pay careful attention to your intake.

Before you start taking supplements, however, try getting more iron in your diet. To reach the recommended amount, which is 10 milligrams for men, 15 milligrams for women age 50 and under, and 10 milligrams for women over 50, consume iron from a variety of sources. Meat is your best source because it contains heme iron, which is the most readily absorbable form. Other good sources of iron are fortified cereals, lentils, and broccoli. Eat a food that is rich in vitamin C, such as strawberries or bell peppers, with your iron source because vitamin C significantly improves iron absorption.

My recommendation: Stay away from supplements that contain more than 15 milligrams of iron. Too much iron can hamper your zinc absorption, making you just as tired as if you had low iron.

Magnesium

For years, researchers have known that magnesium plays a critical role in endurance performance. Magnesium exists mainly inside the cells of muscles and bones, where it assists with muscle contractions and energy metabolism. Studies with lab animals and people show that magnesium deficiency reduces endurance, and that low blood levels of magnesium are associated with decreased aerobic capacity. Unfortunately, extreme endurance events such as marathons can deplete magnesium from your body.

Researchers believe that low magnesium levels reduce production of a substance called 2,3-DPG (or just DPG), which is essential for delivering oxygen to exercising muscles. Theoretically, increasing your magnesium intake will boost your DPG level, thereby improving oxygen delivery and in turn boosting aerobic capacity and performance.

A study done at Lenox Hill Hospital in New York City tested this magnesium-DPG connection with trained runners, who took either a magnesium supplement (at two times the DV) or a placebo for 2 weeks. Runners were tested on the treadmill before and after supplementation. The results showed that the extra magnesium failed to boost circulating DPG level or max VO_2 (the maximum amount of oxygen that can be removed from circulating blood and used by your working tissues during a specified period), and there was no difference in perceived exertion.

The magnesium supplementation may have been superfluous in this case, since the male runners' diets already contained more than the DV of 400 milligrams of magnesium. In other words, more does not mean better.

My recommendation: Try to get your magnesium from food sources such as nuts, molasses, whole grains, and dark green, leafy vegetables because oversupplementation can cause diarrhea and can interfere with calcium absorption and metabolism.

Phytochemicals

Technically, phytochemicals aren't considered nutrients, but these little disease-fighting dynamos are so essential for optimum health that I didn't want to leave them off the list. Found in fruits, vegetables, and grains, there are about 500 different phytochemicals that help protect you against cancer, heart disease, arthritis, and even wrinkles. Researchers are busily isolating these substances—with complicated names such as lycopene and genistein—for companies to sell in pill form.

My recommendation: The best way to fill up on phytochemicals is to eat a variety of fruits, vegetables, and whole grains. No one phytochemical acts as the fountain of youth, and no one food—and especially no one supplement—contains all the phytochemicals. Don't get into a rut of always eating broccoli as your vegetable and an apple as your fruit. Try a new fruit or vegetable each week for variety and better health.

Protein

Every part of your body contains protein, from your muscles and blood and immune cells to your tendons, ligaments, skin, and hair. Sedentary people need 50 to 70 grams of protein a day to keep them going. Fit people need 25 to 50 percent more to take care of muscle repair and increased energy requirements.

The dilemma with protein is that the very people who need more of it, such as endurance exercisers, are often the ones who don't get enough because they tend to eat less meat than sedentary people and bodybuilders, and meat is one of the best sources of protein.

Skimping on protein can cause fatigue and slow recovery from injuries and infections, so be sure you're getting enough from high-quality sources such as lean meat, soybeans (in the form of tofu, soy milk, or soy protein), fish, and low-fat dairy products.

My recommendation: Each day, try to include 5 to 6 ounces of lean meat or two to three servings of soy products, plus two to three servings of low-fat or fat-free dairy products, and several servings of grains along with legumes (especially if you're a vegan). Unless you're a vegan who is allergic to soy, you probably don't need to supplement with protein shakes or energy bars.

Pyruvate

The claims on bottles of pyruvate are stunning: "Increases endurance by 20 percent" and "Promotes 47 percent greater fat loss." According to studies, pyruvate taken in fairly hefty doses of 20 to 25 grams daily appears to boost endurance performance and assist in weight loss. But before you rush out and buy a bottle, read on.

In one study, pyruvate taken on a daily basis boosted endurance in a group of men riding stationary bikes. This may sound promising, but it's important to point out that these men did not exercise regularly and so these results may not apply to people who exercise on a regular basis.

Pyruvate may, however, show more promise as a fat burner. In a study done at the University of Memphis in Tennessee, exercise physiologist Rick Kreider, Ph.D., compared the effects of a daily 10-gram dose of pyruvate to those of a placebo in a group of sedentary, obese women who were beginning a 6-week walking and weight-lifting program. The women lifted weights and walked three times a week for 30 minutes at a time. The women taking the placebo lost no weight over the 6 weeks, while the women who took the pyruvate supplement lost about 1 pound of fat.

"There may be a benefit to taking pyruvate, perhaps at higher doses than used in this experiment," Dr. Kreider notes. "But more research needs to be done, particularly since we found such a small benefit of pyruvate on weight loss. It's also difficult at this point to justify the expense of this supplement, which is about $10 a day." The dosage used in the studies was 15 to 30 times more than what's recommended on product labels.

Meanwhile, Dr. Kreider's colleague, exercise physiologist Pauline Koh, M.S., monitored the women's cholesterol levels during the exercise program. Surprisingly, those taking the pyruvate suffered a drop in levels of HDL (good) cholesterol. And since exercise should boost HDL levels, this ill effect warrants some caution. "While more research is needed to support our work, these results are certainly not desirable for those interested in becoming fit as well as those hoping to ward off heart disease," says Koh.

My recommendation: Thus far, research showing any promise for pyruvate as a fat burner involves daily doses that greatly exceed recommended dosages printed on most product labels. Manufacturers recommend approximately a 1- to 2-gram daily dose. "There's no evidence that pyruvate works in any way at such low levels," says Dr. Kreider. A dosage high enough to be effective would be prohibitively expensive. Don't bother.

Sodium Bicarbonate

There may be something here—if you're a sprinter. Taking a few spoonfuls of sodium bicarbonate (commonly known as baking soda) several hours before a brief but intense bout of exercise may improve your staying power. That's because sodium bicarbonate acts as a buffer in the body, so it decreases lactic acid levels.

Here's how it works. During high-intensity (anaerobic) exercise such as sprinting, your body uses pure carbohydrate—no fat—as a fuel source. A by-product of anaerobic exercise is lactic acid, which is normally cleared away and subsequently used as an energy source itself. If your body produces lactic acid faster than it clears it, the acid begins to hamper muscle contractions, and you get that heavy feeling in your legs.

Several studies have shown that a dose of sodium bicarbonate can delay that feeling, improving performance during short bouts of exercise. But would a shot of sodium bicarbonate before a longer, yet still intense, session of exercise—a 5-K run, for instance—give you an edge?

Researchers from the University of Kansas in Lawrence tested this hypothesis on runners. Each was given 20 grams of sodium bicarbonate 2 hours before an intense 30-minute treadmill run. At the end of the run, the runners sprinted to exhaustion, simulating a finishing kick in a race. The runners gained no benefit from the supplementation, as they sprinted for the same length of time as did a placebo group. One thing this experiment did show is that something other than lactic acid buildup contributes to end-of-race fatigue.

My recommendation: Sodium bicarbonate's fatigue-busting powers come into play only for short-duration, high-intensity exercise, such as sprinting. And beware: Large doses (20 grams or more) of sodium bicarbonate may cause severe intestinal cramping, bloating, and diarrhea, so use it sparingly and only for sprint-type exercise.

Vitamin C

Vitamin C helps protect your body from oxidative damage caused by exercise and other stresses such as air pollution and secondhand smoke. Vitamin C is also critical for maintaining a strong immune system, which can be taxed by endurance exercise.

In a study done at the University of Cape Town Medical School in South Africa, runners took either 600 milligrams of vitamin C a day (10 times the DV) or a placebo for the 3 weeks before an ultramarathon. After the race, the runners who took vitamin C had fewer upper respiratory tract infections than the runners who took a placebo.

My recommendation: Get most of your vitamin C from food. For example, an orange and a kiwifruit each supply close to 100 percent of the DV. Many other fruits and vegetables, such as strawberries, green peppers, and tomatoes, contain more than 50 percent of the DV per serving. If you take supplements, keep your intake below 2,000 milligrams because anything above that level may increase your risk for kidney stones.

Vitamin E

Many researchers believe that the powerful antioxidant properties of vitamin E protect us from the age-related aspects of ailments such as heart disease and cancer. Studies also show that vitamin E supplementation—often at the level of about 400 IU a day—may help protect you from the oxidative damage caused by endurance exercise. This free radical–induced damage is what, in part, causes muscle stiffness and soreness.

I'd love to say that you can get all of the E you need from foods, but that's very difficult to do, especially since 400 IU is more than 1,000 percent of the DV.

My recommendation: Look for a vitamin E supplement that contains no more than 400 IU. Take your supplement with a meal, since your body needs a small amount of fat to break it down. If you'd rather not take a supplement, then the best food sources are almonds and wheat germ; 1 ounce of wheat germ provides 50 percent of your DV. Fortified breakfast cereals are also good choices because they normally contain about 25 percent of the DV.

Whey Protein

A by-product of cheese production, whey protein can supposedly build muscle mass and be absorbed more easily than other proteins. But no research supports such claims.

My recommendation: Until studies find any promise for this supplement, save your money and instead consume your protein from foods such as soy, seafood, eggs, low-fat dairy products, and lean meats.

Zinc

A little zinc goes a long way. Though you have only about 2 grams of it in your body, zinc works in tandem with more than 100 different enzymes, many of which participate in energy metabolism. It's essential for a healthy immune system. It makes wound healing and injury recovery possible, and it's vital for male sexual functioning.

Despite its importance, studies have shown that most people don't consume the DV (15 milligrams) for this mineral. Since you sweat out small amounts of it each time you exercise, you can quickly run the risk of a zinc deficiency. In one study, athletes had twice the zinc loss through urination following a 6-mile run compared to when they didn't exercise.

Up to 40 percent of athletes may have below-normal levels of zinc; a telltale sign of a deficiency is frequent colds. You may also be easily susceptible to infections and bronchitis. Unfortunately, many fit people tend to shy away from the best sources of zinc—oysters, clams, liver, and several kinds of meat—because of the relatively high fat content.

If you're watching the fat in your diet, or if you're a vegetarian, you can get zinc from low-fat foods such as wheat germ, fortified breakfast cereals (they have 25 to 100 percent of the DV per serving), and black-eyed peas, although the zinc found in beef, poultry, pork, lamb, and seafood is absorbed the best.

My recommendation: Supplementation may be the best way to ensure that you get your DV for zinc. Look for a multivitamin/mineral supplement that contains no more than the DV. Remember that high-fiber foods and the tannins found in coffee, some teas, and wine can hamper zinc absorption, so plan your zinc intake accordingly. Also remember that too much zinc blocks the absorption of copper, which in turn impedes iron absorption. You would have to get a lot of zinc to do this, however, since copper deficiency normally results from zinc intakes of six times the DV. You should also know that oversupplementation with zinc has been shown to lower good HDL cholesterol levels and raise harmful LDL cholesterol levels.

part three

Eat to Reach Your Goals

chapter eleven

Lose Weight

I'm proud to say that at age 44, I weigh 120 pounds, which is the same weight I was in college. I'll admit that like most women, perhaps I'm a tad too concerned about my physique. I like to stay trim. I want firm muscles. That's why I swim every morning and cycle most afternoons.

But I've learned through personal experience and my own research that weight control involves more than just exercise. Don't get me wrong, exercise does help. It burns off calories and builds the muscle I need to keep my metabolism supercharged. Plus, all the dieting in the world wouldn't sculpt my arms the way pullups do. Still, I'm sure that if I didn't pay close attention to what I eat, my love affair with chocolate would have padded my frame by now. Getting and staying trim requires a combination of exercise and healthful eating habits.

Food Matters

It seems like there's a new weight-loss guru being interviewed on morning television every week, and the diet gimmick is always different: One week it's grapefruit; the next, steak; the next, a Chinese herb; the next, a liquid fast. All of these diets probably will help you lose weight. What they won't necessarily do is help you take off the pounds in a

workout q&a

Q: Help! I've lost 15 pounds but have hit a plateau. It seems like my metabolism has stopped running. How do I keep losing?

A: Every day, your body spends energy, or calories, to support life-sustaining processes such as keeping your brain switched on. This calorie burning is referred to as your basal metabolic rate (BMR), or your metabolism. Most people burn 800 to 2,000 calories daily to support their BMRs, accounting for most of the calorie needs for the day.

The amount your body spends on your BMR depends upon several factors, including your body size, gender, age, genes, and whether you are a chronic dieter. It's frustrating but true: Your BMR slows down when you cut back on calories. This is a natural protection mechanism that conserves energy so that you don't whittle away to nothing, carried over from when early humans often endured periods with little to eat.

Here's what you can do to get your metabolism burning red-hot.

Add some muscle. Try some strength-building exercise, such as weight training or calisthenics, to build some muscle, which in turn will boost your BMR. Look for a personal trainer certified by the American College of Sports Medicine who can set up a weight-training program that will compliment your aerobic routine.

Boost your exercise time. Twenty to 30 minutes of daily exercise is good, but adding more time or trying new activities, such as bike riding or swimming, will help increase the number of calories you burn.

Rev up your exercise intensity. By picking up your pace, you'll burn extra calories and boost your BMR at the same time. This means that you'll burn some extra calories as your body recovers from exercising.

Waste energy. Your body burns calories when you climb stairs, carry your groceries, do yard work, and simply fidget with your hands. Spend more time on physical activities that you may have avoided with timesaving devices or by hiring someone else to do the work for you.

Eat more. By eating slightly more (since you will be burning more with your increased activity level) you may find you will actually lose weight because your body burns calories while digesting and processing food. Be sure to include several daily servings of fruits and vegetables for extra fiber, which helps you feel full.

healthy manner or help you keep the weight off, so you end up back where you started—looking for a new miracle diet.

It's time to stop the cycle. Gimmick diets make weight loss seem much more complicated than it really is. Simply put, if you want to lose weight, you need to burn more calories than you eat. If you want to keep it off, you can eat only as many calories as you burn.

It sounds simple enough, but few people in the United States do it; we're tempted by supersize portions and calorie-dense processed foods. Most of us eat more fat than we think, and few of us consume enough fruits and vegetables. The combination of all of these factors makes it incredibly difficult to shed pounds. If you don't constantly watch what you eat, all the exercise in the world won't help you lose much weight. Consider the following:

- The average person eats four servings of pasta in a typical restaurant dinner. With tomato sauce, garlic bread, and salad, that comes to more than 1,000 calories. You would have to run 10 miles to burn that many calories through exercise.
- The typical fitness-minded person eats "reward" calories. The thinking goes like this: "Since I just sweated for a half-hour on the stair-stepper, I can have cheesecake for dessert." But the math doesn't work. In a half-hour on a stair-stepper, the typical woman will burn 300 calories at the most. A tiny slice of cheesecake comes to nearly 260 calories. That's fine if you want to hold steady. But it won't help you lose weight.
- Most people who try to lose weight through exercise alone find themselves trapped in a cycle of longer and harder workouts. Eventually, they can't keep up the pace. And when they drop back, they gain weight.

Fortunately, there's a better way, and it doesn't involve liquid fasting, giving up all the foods you love, or feeling constantly starved. By burning off 400 calories on most days and by doing some strength training a couple of days a week, you can rediscover the joy of eating and at the same time get yourself trimmer than you've been in years.

The Anatomy of a Thin Diet

To lose weight and keep it off, you need to make a few simple calculations.

1. **Know how many calories you should be eating.** Most dieters think that they should eat a lot fewer calories than they need to lose weight. Many people tell me about how hard it is to stay on an 800- or 1,000-calorie diet. I always ask, "Why are you trying?" Most people can lose weight on a 1,500- to 2,000-calorie diet.

   Here are the numbers to prove it. To find out how many calories you burn in a day, take your current weight and multiply it by 10. For example, if you weigh 140 pounds, your first number is 1,400. Then add half of your weight to that number. So for our 140-pound person, we end up with 1,470. That's the number of calories you burn every day to breathe, pump blood, and hold a pen at work.

   Now add the number of calories you burn a day during purposeful exercise. I'm asking you to burn 400 calories, which brings the number to 1,870. That's how many calories you need to eat to maintain your weight, assuming you have little muscle mass. (If you've been weight training for a while, add 150 calories). To lose weight, subtract 200 to 500 calories from that number (200 calo-

My Food Diary

I'm a certified chocoholic. During my younger, more naive days, I thought I could overcome my cocoa cravings. I promised myself that I'd eat chocolate only on weekends, or not at all, but it never worked. I would last for a few days, but as soon as I sniffed out the stuff in a coworker's office, at the grocery store, or in my kid's book bag, I would fall off the wagon. And those few days when I did go without chocolate were not pleasant ones for anyone who had to deal with my bad temper.

Now, I eat some chocolate just about every day. My chocolate fix consists of chunks of dark chocolate dipped in peanut butter. I don't even try to make it low-fat or low-calorie; I indulge. Sometimes I'm not in the mood, and on those days, I pass. But those days are few and *very* far between.

I've learned that I need these regular chocolate indulgences to stay satisfied, so I eat my favorite treat without guilt.

ries will be an easier diet to main-tain, while 500 calories will drop the pounds faster; the choice is yours).

2. Know what you're eating. Most di-eters think that they are eating less than they really are. You may hate the idea of keeping a food diary, but I'm asking you to do it only 1 day a week. Write down what you eat, then read the labels of these foods and note the por-tion sizes. For instance, most peo-ple eat 2½ servings at one sitting. Even the bottle of iced tea you drink at lunch has 2 servings. Whether you help yourself or serv-ings are portioned out for you, knowing what counts as 1 serving is important to avoid overeating.

Here are some standard serv-ing sizes. Meats (fish, chicken, beef): 3 ounces cooked, or about the size of a deck of cards. Pasta and other starches: ½ cup cooked (the size of a pudgy computer mouse). Bread: one slice. Mixed entreés, such as casseroles and combination foods: 1 cup (a little bigger than a baseball).

3. Decide what food you really love. Whatever it might be, don't deprive yourself; eat a controlled portion of this food every day. For example, if you love ice cream, eat ½ cup every night for dessert—but eat it slowly, with a small spoon. And get all of those other naughty foods out of your house. Nothing stops mindless munching faster than having no junk food in the house.

4. Keep yourself full with healthy foods. Hunger is one of the worst enemies of a well-intentioned diet, so don't let it happen.

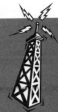

Nutrition News Flash

You've probably heard all of the sta-tistics that say 95 percent of those who lose weight gain it all back within 5 years. I have wonderful news: Those de-pressing statistics are wrong. A study from the University of Pittsburgh Med-ical Center found that nearly 30 percent of those surveyed had lost 10 percent of their body weight and kept it off for more than 5 years.

The results differed because past studies looked only at people who were yo-yo dieters. These people already had the cards stacked against them. The Uni-versity of Pittsburgh Medical Center study looked at a population that more closely resembles the average fitness enthusiast.

Tame Your Hunger

One of the toughest parts of losing weight is getting used to eating less food. We eat for many reasons, including boredom, hunger, sadness, and stress. Whenever you have the urge to eat, first ask yourself why you are eating. If you really are hungry, go ahead. But if you're not truly hungry, find another way to deal with your emotions.

If you feel hungry all day long, you can tame those stomach rumblings by following these strategies.

Eat a big breakfast. Studies show that people who eat a high-carbohydrate breakfast and lunch end up eating more calories and fat later in the afternoon than people who fuel up earlier in the day with a large meal that contains a balance of carbohydrate, fat, and protein. This is contrary to the way most people eat when they're dieting. Most people don't eat much in the morning and then end up bingeing in the afternoon and evening. And they don't even realize that they're doing it to themselves.

Fuel up with a 600-calorie breakfast and then have a protein-rich mid-morning snack. Most people don't even come close to 600 calories at breakfast; the typical bowl of cereal and milk supplies only 250 to 300 calories. Remember that you want a combination of carbohydrate, protein, and fat. Scrambled eggs with toast and peanut butter, for instance, will keep you full throughout the morning and prevent you from overindulging in something fatty later in the day.

Never skip a meal. People who exercise need to eat every 3 to 4 hours. That may sound like a lot, but it's the only way you can control your hunger and keep yourself from bingeing. And it's the only way to keep your metabolism moving.

Studies of gymnasts and soccer players show exactly how dramatically calorie deprivation can bring your metabolism to a screeching halt. Researchers learned that the gymnasts were barely surviving on 800 calories a day while the soccer players were eating 3,000 calories. But the soccer players burned more than three times as many calories as the gymnasts. That wasn't because the soccer players were working out that much harder, it was because the chronic calorie deprivation of the gymnasts had slowed their metabolisms. Whenever your body thinks that it will not get food, it slows your metabolism to compensate.

Recipe Revver

Appetite-Control Minestrone Soup
Serves a family of four for a week

With an abundance of veggies, this filling soup has only about 200 calories per big bowl.

     2   beef shanks (about 2 pounds), optional
     1   tablespoon canola oil (optional)
    10   cups water
     1   bay leaf
     1   large onion, chopped
     3   cloves garlic, minced
     5   large ribs celery, chopped
     1   can (15 ounces) tomato sauce
     1   can (15 ounces) kidney beans, rinsed and drained
     1   can (15 ounces) lima beans, rinsed and drained
     1   can (15 ounces) chickpeas, rinsed and drained
    ¾   cup chopped carrots
    ¾   cup chopped green beans
    ¾   cup corn
    ¾   cup chopped okra
     2   cups small, shaped pasta
   1–3   tablespoons pesto
         Salt and pepper
         Freshly grated Parmesan cheese, for sprinkling

In a large soup pot, sear the meat in the canola oil for 5 minutes (if using). Add the water and bay leaf to the pot and bring to a boil. Simmer for 1½ hours. Add the onion, garlic, celery, and tomato sauce. Simmer for another hour. Add the kidney and lima beans, chickpeas, carrots, green beans, corn, and okra. Simmer for another 15 minutes. Add the pasta and simmer another 10 minutes, or until the pasta is tender. Season to taste with the pesto, salt, and pepper. Remove and discard the bay leaf. Ladle the soup into serving bowls and sprinkle with the cheese.

Per 2-cup serving: 238 calories, 17 g protein, 29 g carbohydrate, 6 g total fat, 2 g saturated fat, 20 mg cholesterol, 5.5 g dietary fiber, 194 mg sodium

You're not going to be eating huge meals every 3 to 4 hours. You need to hold your total daily calories to your predetermined goal, so feed yourself mini meals.

Start with soup. Studies done at Pennsylvania State University in University Park show that foods with a high water content are most filling. Soup is the best example. Try to have soup every night for dinner as your first course. Make it a chunky, broth-based type and eat as much as you want. An entire large jar of soup has only 300 calories. Once you're done with your soup, you can eat more—if you're still hungry.

Reach for vegetables and fruit. Aim for at least eight servings of fruits and vegetables daily. A serving equals one medium-size fruit (about the size of a tennis ball), 1 cup raw, ½ cup cooked, or 4 ounces of juice. At lunch and dinner, make the most of your salad by including a variety of dark green lettuces, fresh cut vegetables, beans, and sprouts topped off with 1 to 2 tablespoons of oil and vinegar dressing or just plain vinegar. Fruits and vegetables fill you up and may keep you from going back for seconds of tacos, pizza, or desserts.

Eat heavy foods. Appetite-control researchers have found that your brain may monitor how much to eat based on the weight of your food. While munching on a bag of potato chips, you can easily chomp down 300 calories in a few handfuls and still feel hungry. But have you ever tried eating 300 calories worth of oranges in one sitting? That's five whole ones, to be exact. Regardless of the calories or fat they contain, lightweight foods such as chips, crackers, rice cakes, and popcorn don't satisfy your hunger as well as heavier foods such as fruits and vegetables do.

In a study done at the University of Auckland in New Zealand, people automatically stopped eating when they had consumed a particular weight of food, regardless of the amount of fat and calories. If the food was light but high in calories, they could easily consume 1,000 calories or more and not feel stuffed. But they stopped eating heavy low-calorie foods after just a few hundred calories.

Fruits and vegetables are your best bet. For desserts, try pumpkin pie or hot chocolate instead of German chocolate cake or Boston cream pie. Also, eat fewer lightweight, calorie-dense munchies like chips, cheese puffs, candy, and crackers. Desserts to avoid include cheesecake, whipped cream, and fudge.

Limit your choices. According to anthropologists, we are programmed to eat more when we're offered choices. Perhaps this is a throwback to our cave-dwelling ancestors, who wouldn't have survived if they hadn't eaten a variety of nuts, berries, and wild animals.

A study done at Tufts University in Medford, Massachusetts, found that people who eat the widest variety of certain types of food (especially sweets, pizza, and sandwiches) have more body fat than those who stick with just one type of dessert or other high-calorie fare. Today, people eat more calories for dessert when they are offered cookies, cheesecake, pudding, and other choices than when they are offered only cheesecake. On the other hand, people who eat the widest variety of fruits and vegetables have slightly less body fat than those who eat the same two or three produce items all the time.

Allow yourself just one selection of a particular type of food. For example, have only one appetizer, one side dish, one main dish, one dessert item, and one beverage when eating out. At home, stock only one type of a high-calorie item. For example, buy only one ice cream flavor or one brand of soda. You'll automatically eat less but still feel satisfied.

Think small. Our cave-dwelling relatives didn't know when their next meal was coming, so they had to devour everything they could get their hands on to survive. Today, food is much less scarce, but we still tend to eat everything we see. You can block that primitive urge to overeat simply by offering yourself smaller portions. Start by taking the smallest plate available, which will help make portions appear larger. Also, dish up petite servings—a dab of this and a pinch of that. You'll spare yourself unwanted calories but still taste the foods you love.

Move before munching. Slip in a quick, vigorous workout before you go to a party or restaurant. In one study, a group of cyclists pedaled briskly on a stationary bike for 30 minutes while another group pedaled slowly. A third group didn't exercise at all. When offered food 15 minutes later, the fast-pedaling cyclists weren't hungry and initially turned the food away, while the slower cyclists and nonexercisers dug in.

Drink before dining. In one study, people who ran on a treadmill for 50 minutes and then drank some water ate fewer calories later in the day than people who drank either a sugar-sweetened or artificially flavored, zero-calorie beverage. Something about the sweet taste of a drink (even a diet drink) can prime your stomach to crave more food, but plain water reduces your hunger.

Smell your food. Research shows that people who focus on eating by taking small bites, chewing thoroughly, and paying more attention to smell and taste eat fewer calories than those who do not. Pay close attention to taste. Once what you're eating no longer tastes as delicious as when you started, stop eating. That's a subtle but important cue from your stomach to your mouth that you've eaten enough calories.

Limit your liquid calories. Typical beverages, especially alcoholic ones, are laden with calories that don't fill you up. Fruit juice, punch, soda, wine, beer, liquor, and champagne contain 150 or more calories per 8 ounces. Several drinks (with or without alcohol) can amount to 600 to 800 calories. Try to cut back on these liquid calories as much as you can by switching to sparkling water. Add some fresh mint leaves and cranberries to the glass for some flavor and a touch of festivity.

Be smart with sweets. If you really love chocolate, pie, or cookies, don't try to do without them. Cutting sweets out completely, even for 1 to 2 days, can set off a sugar binge. It's best to indulge in frequent but small servings. When buying sweets, look for bite-size or single-serving packages so that it's not a big deal if you eat the whole thing. And eat sweets with your meals instead of making snacking a special event. This helps keep serving sizes small.

Holiday Helper

Festive times of the year are more challenging when it comes to controlling your urge to eat. Here are tips for handling your hunger in some particularly difficult situations.

Parties

- Eat something before arriving at a party. A ravenous, hollow stomach will lead to out-of-control eating.

- Position yourself away from the food table. That will allow you to visit with the other partygoers and not focus on the food.
- Survey the food table quickly and start off with some fresh vegetables or fruit.
- When selecting items that you know are higher in calories and fat, ask yourself if this food is unique or special for the holidays. You can eat a handful of chocolate candies at any time of the year, but a distinctive appetizer or cookie may be more worth a nibble right now.
- Ask the host beforehand if you can contribute to the party goodies. Suggest fresh vegetables with salsa, or hummus dip with whole grain pita slices.
- If you are going to more than one party in an evening, pace yourself. Eating is not a must for celebrating.

Holiday Meals

- If you're not the cook, get some exercise just before the big feast. Studies show that exercising just before eating may suppress the appetite.
- Avoid skipping meals beforehand so that you can rationalize the "big" meal. Banking calories for later in the day may make you ravenously hungry and lead to overeating.
- If possible, eat your large meal in the afternoon, which gives your body time to comfortably digest the food and may leave you time for physical activity, such as an evening walk.
- Serve yourself smaller portions—you can always go back for more. Assure the cook that your smaller portions allow you to savor every bite. It also helps you rationalize having seconds of your favorites.
- Allow yourself 15 to 20 minutes to rest before you reach for seconds. That will give your stomach time to signal your brain that you've had enough.
- Fill your plate with low-fat items first, such as steamed vegetables, sweet potatoes, salads (go easy on the dressing), or lean meats, including skinless turkey or low-fat ham.
- Sip flavored coffees (hazelnut, chocolate, vanilla) before dessert. Their sweet taste may satisfy your desire for after-dinner sweets.

Giving Food Gifts

- Give a colorful array of dried fruits (peaches, apricots, persimmons, papayas, apples) and nuts (walnuts, almonds, hazelnuts, pecans) instead of calorie-laden cookies and candies.
- A live herb plant for a window garden or a selection of herb seeds makes a great gift for a gardener-chef.
- A sampling of flavored mustards—garlic, chili, or herb—is wonderful for spicing up soups, sandwiches, and salads.
- Give a kitchen gadget that brings good health, such as one of those big soft-grip vegetable peelers or garlic presses. A vegetable brush makes a good gift for that friend who avoids veggies because of the hassle it takes to prepare them.
- Put together a selection of beans (kidneys, lentils) along with seasonings and other ingredients and give it with your favorite chili or soup recipe for a very personal gift.

Gain Weight

Many people in American society are preoccupied with images of big thighs, potbellies, and flabby rear ends. Yet for those people with "scrawny" arms and "stick" legs, the battle to gain weight can be just as frustrating as the struggle for those who want to lose it.

I often hear from men who want to "beef up," particularly those interested in adding muscle. But some women also struggle with trying to add more weight, particularly taller women, who tend to burn more calories as a result of their height.

Why are you so skinny while everyone around you seems to be dieting? You can blame it on your parents, grandparents, and great grandparents, who most likely all were slender. Your genetics may go a long way toward keeping the weight off, but that doesn't mean you should give up hope. Once you combine strategic eating with a quality strength-training program, you can put on weight and feel great.

Food Is Your Friend

To encourage your body to hold on to calories instead of burn them, take the following steps.

Consume extra calories. Women need 20 to 22 calories per pound of body weight; men need 23 or more calories. If you weigh 130 pounds, your

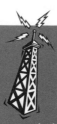

Nutrition News Flash

We used to think that eggs were bad for your heart because they're high in cholesterol. But research has failed to strongly link dietary cholesterol with blood cholesterol. A study published in the *Journal of the American Medical Association* comparing egg eaters to non–egg eaters found that people who ate an egg every single day had no increase in their risk for heart disease.

math would look like this: 22 calories per pound × 130 pounds = 2,860 calories a day. This is 500 to 800 calories more than your regular caloric needs. At this rate of intake, you should be able to put on about ½ pound per week.

Eat enough protein. Most people who want to gain weight don't want to gain just any weight. They want to build muscle, tissue which requires protein. Studies show that weight lifting and other vigorous exercise like running, cycling, and team sports boost protein needs an estimated 50 percent or more above the Daily Value (DV).

You need 90 to 100 grams of protein daily, or about 0.7 gram for every pound of body weight. If you weigh 150 pounds, you should be eating 90 to 130 grams of protein a day. You can easily meet these protein needs by eating foods such as canned tuna, tofu, eggs, chicken, and lean meats.

Focus on quality. Your body needs vitamins, minerals, and essential fats for weight gain (not to mention for good health). You get all of these nutrients from eating wholesome foods such as whole grains, fruits, and vegetables. You may want to consider taking a multivitamin/mineral supplement to fill in the gaps.

The Specifics

Eating more protein and more calories sounds simple—until you try it. Then you realize that the more you try to stuff yourself with food, the less you feel like eating. Here are some tips to make eating less of a chore.

Don't ever skip a meal. Eat a hearty breakfast, lunch, and dinner plus at least two snacks (one before bedtime). If you eat every few hours, you will be able to consume those extra calories without feeling stuffed. If you tend to get heartburn when you eat close to bedtime, have your snack a couple of hours before you hit the sack.

Beef up your portions. Add more cereal to your bowl in the morning, pile on more sandwich fillings at lunch, and serve yourself a generous portion of potatoes at dinner. By eating larger servings, you can sneak in extra calories.

Eat calorie-rich foods. Add high-calorie foods such as ice cream, nuts, peanut butter, and applesauce to your diet. Go ahead and slather peanut butter on a whole grain bagel, dip your chips in guacamole, or drink fruit juices instead of water or diet drinks. (Just one bottle of fruit juice can yield up to 400 calories.) When choosing cereals, opt for higher-calorie granola-and-nut mixes rather than lower-calorie airy puffs. Don't shy away from the occasional beer along with some nuts and chips. And consider meal-supplement drinks such as Ensure or Boost, which also supply plenty of calories.

Profiling Protein

Just because you need added protein to gain weight doesn't mean you have to take supplements. Here's a look at how much protein you need, how you can get it, and the risks you face if you consume too much.

Your protein requirement is based on your body weight. The DV for protein is 0.36 gram per pound of body weight—that's almost 65 grams for a person who weighs 180 pounds. But the extra 50 percent needed by people who play hard bumps the requirement up to 125 grams daily for a 180-pound athlete. Your body uses the extra protein for building and repairing muscle tissue and also burns a small amount for fuel.

Eating more than 100 grams of protein daily may sound challenging, but there's a good chance that you already get this much from food alone. Most of the athletes I work with easily meet their increased protein needs by eating foods such as fish, lean meats, soy, eggs, beans, and dairy products. (A 3-ounce serving of fish or lean meat has 21 grams of protein.) The only athletes who fall short of their protein requirements are those who omit high-protein foods like meat and eggs and who don't compensate for that protein deficit somewhere else in their diets.

Even if you are a vegetarian, supplementation probably isn't neces-

Recipe Revver

High-Protein Smoothie
Makes 1

This smoothie contains no supplements or powders. Rather, it has 100 percent wholesome ingredients and is loaded with vitamins C, and B$_6$, antioxidants, potassium, and fiber. And because the liquid egg substitute is pasteurized, it's safe to eat raw.

  1 *cup ice cubes*
  ¾ *cup pasteurized liquid egg substitute*
  ¾ *cup vanilla soy milk*
  1 *cup frozen blueberries*
  ½ *banana, sliced*
  ½ *cup cranberry juice*
  1 *tablespoon honey*

In a blender, combine the ice, egg substitute, milk, blueberries, banana, juice, and honey. Process on high for 30 seconds. Pour into a tall glass.

Per smoothie: *400 calories, 5 g total fat, 25 g protein, 65 g carbohydrate, 5.5 g dietary fiber, 0 mg cholesterol, 489 sodium*

sary. Most supplements are derived from soy or milk, which are great natural sources of protein that your body processes very efficiently. Sure, you can ingest your protein in supplement form, but you can get the same amount for less money from a tofu stir-fry or a carton of soy milk.

Some of the athletes I counsel prefer protein powder supplements as a matter of convenience. These athletes often don't have time to prepare their own meals, so using a supplement helps them get the protein that their bodies need. If you live on a diet of convenience foods, these powders may be beneficial. You can add them to fruit smoothies, soups, and casseroles. Most powder supplements provide 15 to 30 grams of protein per serving. Check the label of your product to see how much protein it contains.

Be careful, however, because you can easily consume more protein than your body needs, and for some people, this may be risky. Your kidneys process the extra protein, and then your body burns it as fuel or converts it to fat and stores it for later use. People with kidney disease should avoid extra protein. If you have a history of kidney disease in your family, talk to your doctor before adding any type of protein supplement to your diet.

Will Creatine Help?

Creatine has become a hot-selling supplement among athletes, and for good reason. In certain situations, a dose of creatine will improve muscle strength, boost speed, and may even help increase muscle mass.

Creatine is a proteinlike substance that your body makes on a daily basis; you also get it from your diet if you eat beef, fish, and other meats. If you're a vegetarian and get your protein from milk, eggs, tofu, and beans, you don't get any creatine in your diet. That's okay because you make all you need for typical body functions.

Creatine's most notable activity takes place in your muscle tissue. It acts much like the cylinders in your car's engine, helping to fire up your muscles during high-intensity exercise such as weight lifting, jumping, or sprinting. If you take a creatine supplement of 20 to 25 grams for 5 to 7 days, you'll boost the number of cylinders (creatine levels) in your muscles by 20 to 30 percent. As a result, you'll have a greater ability to do single or repeated bouts of high-intensity exercise such as sprinting or (more important for beefing up) bench-pressing.

When taken over several weeks, reports show that creatine can help build muscle size when you combine supplementation with a strength-training program. In a study from Truman State University in Kirksville, Missouri, men who weight trained took creatine for 6 weeks and experienced significant gains in lean tissue—approximately 4 pounds—compared to men who took a placebo.

But before you take this as a green light to start supplementation, there are some issues to consider. Not everyone gets the same magnitude of benefit from creatine supplements. Some studies show minimal (if any) gains in muscle mass. And research has not been performed on younger athletes, especially adolescents who are still growing.

workout q&a

Q: I'm a woman who can't seem to get any muscle definition. Help!

A: About a quarter of a woman's body weight is fat, and much of it is stored in places such as the breasts, hips, thighs, and butt. These fat-storage sites are considered crucial for reproduction because fat provides fuel for normal menstrual cycles, pregnancy, and breastfeeding. Women also tend to carry more of their body fat underneath the skin. This subcutaneous fat covers the muscles, giving women a smooth appearance.

Men have less subcutaneous fat, so there's often little more than skin resting over their muscles, especially if their overall body fat levels are low. As a result, men typically have more muscle definition, especially on their arms and legs. The sex hormones estrogen and testosterone are primarily responsible for this visual effect.

Female bodybuilders who take the male hormone testosterone (also called an anabolic steroid) can achieve the masculine appearance of muscle definition. But taking these steroids (or other performance-enhancing drugs) can have serious and even deadly health consequences.

Despite the hope and the claims that you can alter any and every aspect of your body "for the better," the fact is that you were born with a body type that you cannot change. Determined by genetics, your body type may tend toward one or another of the three categories established by American psychologist W. H. Sheldon in the 1930s. (The "average" person has an equal mix of all three.)

Ectomorph: Thin, slender hips, not well-muscled

Endomorph: Round, pear-shape body with a smooth look as a result of a higher fat-to-muscle ratio

Mesomorph: Broad shoulders, hourglass shape, higher muscle-to-fat ratio

Unless you lose weight or undergo liposuction, you may not have a good chance of seeing muscle definition. If you increase the amount of weight you are lifting, you may get more muscle definition, but you'll most likely get an increase in bulk, too.

Your natural body type is yours to make the most of and enjoy, so continue exercising and varying your weight-lifting exercises every several weeks to develop and tone the different muscle groups.

The long-term safety of creatine has not been adequately explored. A few studies have looked at the medical safety of taking standard doses of creatine over several weeks. One study showed that supplementing with creatine did not alter liver and kidney function, which is a good sign because these two organs are involved with clearing creatine from the body.

Muscle cramping may be a possible side effect of creatine supplementation. Many athletes have told me that they've experienced muscle cramping during training and even during competition. When they stop taking creatine for several days, the cramping stops. But only a few studies have confirmed this problem. One suspicion is that the extra water retention in the muscle tissue may interfere with proper muscle contraction, causing the cramping.

Even putting these possible safety issues aside, the news about the lasting power of creatine is discouraging. Once you stop taking creatine, the performance benefits disappear. And researchers don't know what may happen to your body's ability to make creatine if you stay on supplements for an extended period of time. Considering that creatine supplements are fairly expensive, the temporary boost hardly seems worth it. Personally, I am a firm believer in doing the best with what you have.

In the Weight Room

In addition to eating the extra food it takes to put on weight, you also need to exercise to avoid gaining weight in your fat cells. You want to beef up your arms and legs by adding muscle, which takes strength training. If you've never strength trained before, find an experienced personal trainer certified by the American College of Sports Medicine who can get you started.

Develop a program that consists of 8 to 10 different weight-lifting exercises that target the major muscle groups in your body, such as the chest, legs, back, arms, and belly. At minimum, you should perform each exercise in a set of 10 to 15 repetitions, or reps for short. And you should lift weights two or three times per week.

The best approach to building muscle is to work up to lifting three sets of 10 to 15 reps for each of the different exercises. Three sets may

Eating Smart for...
Beefing Up

This day of high-quality eating will give you an extra 500 to 1,000 calories, depending on your body size and exercise level.

Breakfast
Two eggs (or 4 ounces liquid egg substitute) scrambled with 1 ounce diced ham and 1 ounce grated Cheddar cheese

One whole wheat bagel spread with 2 tablespoons peanut butter

1 cup fruit salad

8 ounces orange-mango fruit juice

Morning Snack
One pita filled with 2 tablespoons hummus and cucumber slices

8 ounces 1% milk

Lunch
Turkey sandwich (two hefty slices whole grain bread, 3 ounces roasted turkey, 1 ounce provolone cheese, one-eighth avocado)

One banana

Two chocolate-chip cookies

8 ounces cranberry juice

Afternoon Snack
2 ounces trail mix (peanuts, raisins, dried coconut)

2 ounces pretzel sticks dipped in 1 cup chocolate pudding

8 ounces vanilla soy milk

Dinner
4 ounces grilled fish over 1½ cups risotto

1 cup steamed broccoli with 1 tablespoon grated Parmesan cheese

2 cups salad made with your choice of veggies, ½ ounce goat cheese, ½ ounce roasted almonds, and 1 tablespoon olive oil dressing

1 whole grain roll with 2 teaspoons trans-free margarine

Evening Snack
One slice of berry pie topped with ice cream

Calories: 3,700; Protein: 150 grams; Carbohydrate: 458 grams; Fat: 33% calories

sound like a lot, but once you get your program going, it should take only 30 to 40 minutes per session. You may read some books that tell you that one set is all you need to do, and that's fine if you're looking for just a little muscle definition. But if you are planning to build a larger amount of muscle, you need more than one set to accomplish your goal, especially after you get through the first few months of weight lifting, when your strength tends to increase quickly and then reaches a plateau.

In addition to lifting multiple sets, you must use a weight that completely fatigues you in 10 to 15 reps. If you lift a weight that is too light, you'll be wasting your time in the gym.

For the Terminally Thin

Some thin individuals struggle to gain weight even with the best programs. Because of their genes, they have a difficult time putting on pounds no matter what.

Keep in mind that adding quality weight takes patience and time. But if you still have trouble beefing up, try increasing your intake by another 500 to 750 calories daily. You could also add more fat to your diet to increase calorie density. In this way, you will be able to eat more. Add snacks that include nuts, avocados, and peanut butter. Be patient; you should see some results in 5 to 7 weeks.

chapter thirteen

Boost Your Immunity

H aving a cold is no fun. While you certainly can exercise with a cold (moderate physical activity won't make it worse), few people feel like doing so. It's annoying and embarrassing to keep blowing and wiping your nose as you work the pedals of the stair-stepper. Plus, you have about as much energy as Sleeping Beauty.

The common cold may be one of the biggest contributors to the sedentary lifestyle. Many people rev up their fitness programs just after New Year's (health club employees call these people the resolutioners). They show up faithfully for a few weeks and then get socked for a week with a cold or the flu. Once they're out of the habit of exercising, making a trip to the gym becomes that much less likely. Few recovering resolutioners jump back on the exercise wagon.

Steering Clear of Colds

The average adult gets two to four colds each year. Children come down with at least six. While most colds tend to be mild and last about a week, this common illness is the leading cause of physician visits and missed days from work and school.

Fortunately, most fitness enthusiasts have strong immune systems. Studies show that regular, moderate exercise can keep colds and flu at bay. In fact, in a *Runner's World* magazine survey, 61 percent of 700 recreational runners said that they experienced fewer colds after beginning a fitness routine. And when you do catch a cold, it usually doesn't last as long or make you feel as dreadful as it would for someone whose primary form of exercise is pressing the buttons on the TV remote control.

Problems arise, however, when you move beyond moderate exercise to more vigorous endurance exercises such as marathons, triathlons, and century cycling. Studies show that fitness enthusiasts who engage in these kinds of activities are more likely to develop colds, especially during the week after the big event. In one study done after the 1987 Los Angeles Marathon, one out of seven runners caught a cold the week after the race. Both physical and mental stress can lower immunity, making you more susceptible to nasty germs.

Following a tough endurance effort, the most important thing you can do is rest. I suggest taking a weeklong vacation after your marathon or century. After all, you've earned it! The second most important thing you can do is to avoid the germs that could make you sick. Wash your hands obsessively; avoid touching your eyes, nose, or mouth with your hands; stay away from children with runny noses, if possible; and avoid airline flights, where germs tend to circulate in the cabin.

Whether you exercise moderately or intensely, you don't want to let the occasional cold sideline your workout plans. Taking steps to keep your immune system strong year-round is an important part of eating smart.

The Immune System

Your immune system is two-tiered. The outer line of defense includes your skin (washing your hands frequently is one way to prevent infection) and the mucus-lined tissues of your body such as your sinus passages, lungs, and even your intestinal tract. These tissues become more porous if you don't eat healthfully. (Vitamin A is especially important for keeping your tissues less porous.) When that happens, disease-causing bacteria and viruses are free to enter your body.

The second level of defense involves your white blood cells and other killer cells that recognize pathogens inside your body. These specialized

workout q&a

Q: Is it safe to exercise with a cold?

A: Use this age-old advice: If your symptoms are from the neck up, go ahead and work out at a moderate pace. If you feel achy and tired all over—which means that you are probably running a fever—you should rest until you feel better.

cells actually "remember" repeat intruders and destroy them, which is how a vaccination works. But this wonderfully complex system relies on a number of nutrients to function properly. Without an adequate intake of such things as copper, zinc, and protein, you leave yourself open to attack by all kinds of insidious invaders.

Nine Foods That Fend Off Infection

So how do you keep your immune system functioning optimally? Well, the best defense is a good offense. Arm yourself with these nine proven immunity-boosting foods this winter—or anytime.

Almonds

Almonds are an excellent source of vitamin E (so are sunflower seeds and wheat germ). You usually hear that this vitamin can protect you against heart disease and certain cancers, but it also boosts your immunity.

Researchers suspect that our immune systems weaken as we age, leading to more frequent infections and slower recovery from illness. That's where vitamin E comes in. A study of men and women age 65 and older showed that supplementing with vitamin E seemed to halt this decline in immunity. The subjects took either 200 IU of vitamin E or a placebo daily for 7 months. At the end of this period, those who took the supplements showed a better immune response to a vaccine.

A little more than a handful of almonds contains 100 percent of the Daily Value (DV) of vitamin E. Sprinkle some on top of your cereal, mix them into your casseroles, or just munch on them plain. Trying to get 200 IU of vitamin E (20 times the DV) every day in your diet is going to be pretty tough, so you may want to consider a supplement.

Bananas

Eating plenty of bananas will help you get enough vitamin B_6 since one medium banana supplies about 30 percent of the DV. (It also comes with about 100 carbohydrate calories and no fat.) Vitamin B_6 works like this: When an invading virus or bacterium enters your body, certain immune cells recognize the intruder and quickly set out to destroy it. Vitamin B_6 is critical to this recognition process.

Many people don't get enough B_6 because unlike many other B vitamins, it isn't normally added to refined grain products such as bread. That's why bananas are so important. Put them in fruit smoothies, slice them onto your cereal, or eat them plain. Because they are digested so quickly, you can eat them just before or during your workout.

If you don't like bananas, you can get B_6 from potatoes, chickpeas, and chicken breast meat.

Beer and Chocolate

Beer and chocolate are a dynamic duo when it comes to boosting your immune system. Both are high in copper, an important member of

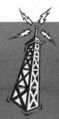

Nutrition News Flash

If you're training for a marathon or century bike ride, learning how to consume calories during your workout can do more than fuel your exercise; it might even keep you from getting sick.

Studies done by renowned immunity researcher David C. Nieman, Ph.D., professor of health and exercise science at Appalachian State University in Boone, North Carolina, has found that consuming small amounts of carbohydrate during endurance exercise can prevent the postexercise drop in immunity that tends to occur after heavy-duty exercise. That's just one more important reason to consume 30 to 60 grams of carbohydrate during every hour of exercise. That comes to 120 to 240 calories per hour.

Recipe Revver

Caribbean Chicken
Serves 4

When I serve this chicken dish over brown rice, I know that my family is getting plenty of vitamin C, protein, and zinc to fight off colds and flu.

- 4 boneless, skinless chicken breast halves
- 1 ripe mango
  Zest and juice of 1 lemon
- ½ cup finely chopped red onion
- 1 small jalapeño pepper, seeded and finely chopped (wear plastic gloves when handling)
- 2 tablespoons honey
  Dash of allspice
  Dash of cinnamon
  Freshly ground black pepper

Preheat the oven to 375°F. Place the chicken in a glass baking dish and set aside. In a medium bowl, mash the mango and combine the lemon zest and juice, onion, jalapeño, honey, allspice, and cinnamon. Mix evenly and season to taste with the black pepper. Spread the mixture over the chicken and cover the baking dish with foil. Bake for 45 minutes, or until a thermometer inserted in the thickest portion registers 160°F and the juices run clear. Uncover and broil for 10 minutes, or until the top is bubbly.

Per serving: 222 calories, 3 g total fat, 1 g saturated fat, 28 g protein, 21 g carbohydrate, 3 g dietary fiber, 73 mg cholesterol, 67 mg sodium

your immunity arsenal. (Nuts, seafood, and beans are also good sources.) Average copper intake is a tough thing to measure, but studies indicate that many of us don't get the recommended 1½ to 5 milligrams a day. That's not good, as studies also show that a chronically low copper intake can weaken your body's disease-fighting cells.

I don't know about you, but that's how I'm going to rationalize keeping chocolate around as a dietary staple.

Butternut Squash

This type of squash is a much appreciated wintertime source of beta-carotene. An antioxidant precursor of vitamin A, beta-carotene keeps your so called killer cells working properly. Beta carotene is also converted into vitamin A in your intestinal tract, and vitamin A helps keep all of your mucous membranes healthy and free from dryness or tiny cracks that could allow foreign matter into your body. Studies clearly show that a deficiency of beta-carotene or vitamin A increases your susceptibility to infection.

Steam or microwave butternut squash, then mash it and serve it as a side dish. Or mix mashed squash with fat-free liquid egg substitute to make beta "pancakes"—a healthful and colorful way to start your day.

Oranges

One orange supplies far more than 100 percent of your daily vitamin C needs. That's good news for your immune system because your skin and other protective tissues need vitamin C to keep them healthy. Vitamin C is also vital to the proper functioning of T cells. Produced in your bone marrow, T cells are lymphocytes that attack pathogens in the bloodstream.

Some reports suggest that it takes much more than the DV of 60 milligrams of vitamin C to decrease your risk of upper respiratory tract infections. Keep a big bowl of oranges on hand all winter and stay well-stocked with other vitamin C–rich fruits (kiwifruits, berries, melons) and vegetables (peppers, broccoli, tomatoes), and aim for seven servings a day of foods rich in vitamin C.

Oysters

Oysters pack a whopping 500 percent of the DV for zinc in a 3-ounce serving, far more than other zinc-rich foods such as meat and beans. This mineral is crucial to the healthy functioning of your body's phagocytes (literally, eating cells). These tough guys engulf foreign bacteria and other invaders, rendering them harmless. Zinc is also essential to another part of your immune system called humural immunity, which works by chemically inactivating incoming bacteria.

Eating Smart for...
Boosting Immunity

This is a typical menu for me during the height of the cold-and-flu season.

Breakfast
1 cup oatmeal topped with 2 tablespoons chopped almonds and 2 tablespoons raisins
One slice whole grain bread
One orange
4 ounces soy milk

Morning Snack
½ cup dried papaya and soy nut mixture
1 cup black tea sweetened with 2 teaspoons honey and lemon

Lunch
1 cup lentil soup (ready-to-eat from a can or dry mix made with hot water)
One 3-inch square of cornbread
10 baby carrots dipped in 3 tablespoons hummus
1 ounce dark chocolate

Afternoon Snack
2 whole grain crackers spread with 1 ounce goat cheese
8 ounces cranberry juice

Dinner
1 serving Caribbean Chicken (see page 154) served over ¾ cup brown rice
2 cups dark, leafy greens
1 cup fruit salad (oranges, pears, peaches)

Calories: 2,000; Protein: 85 grams; Carbohydrate: 320 grams; Fat: 20% calories

Surveys show that most of us don't get enough zinc. To help you consistently hit the DV of 15 milligrams, try to include more oysters in your diet. Add them to casseroles, chowders, and soups.

Tuna

One of the best protein buys around, a can of tuna will give you 22 grams of immunity-boosting protein per 3-ounce serving. You should get

75 to 100 grams of protein a day because fit people need more than sedentary folks. It's especially important to get enough during periods of hard training or racing.

It's well-known that intense training or racing can suppress your immune system. (It's been shown that the risk of colds and upper respiratory infection rises just after a long race.) At these times, protein is diverted for use as energy, so there's less of it for your body to use in manufacturing new immune cells and other substances necessary for defense against infection. That's where tuna (packed in water, not fat-laden oil) can help.

Other good protein sources are lean red meats, poultry, low-fat dairy items, grains, beans, and soy products.

Yogurt

Eat yogurt every day if possible, and be sure to buy the kind that contains live and active cultures. Research suggests that eating 2 cups of live-and-active-culture yogurt each day boosts your body's production of gamma-interferon, a substance that is crucial to your immune system. Studies show that women who eat yogurt daily also have a lower incidence of vaginal yeast infections. Yogurt's active bacterial cultures crowd out harmful bacteria and other unwanted microorganisms.

Use plain yogurt instead of sour cream on baked potatoes, or mix yogurt into sauces to create a creamy texture. Yogurt also makes a great staple for fruit smoothies, and it's perfect as a snack at work.

Common Cures

Once you succumb to a cold or flu, what's your aching body to do? Studies have looked at the use of zinc lozenges or tablets taken several times a day after a cold begins. While a few studies show that the zinc reduced the number of days with cold symptoms, most studies showed no benefit. Also, zinc lozenges resulted in side effects such as a bad taste in the mouth, nausea, and mouth and throat irritation—not what you want along with already uncomfortable cold symptoms.

A delivery system for zinc, however, shows promise in beating back colds and shortening the number of days that your symptoms last. Zinc nasal spray, sold as an over-the-counter product called Zicam, may shorten the life of a cold, according to at least one study. Subjects used either the zinc spray or a placebo within 24 hours of getting cold symptoms and were asked to keep a diary tracking their illnesses. Zinc spray users experienced symptoms for a mere 1½ days compared to 10 days for subjects using the placebo nasal spray. More studies are needed to verify these results and to determine whether children can safely use zinc sprays.

The debate over the vitamin C connection to curing colds has been running like a drippy nose since the 1970s. Many studies have shown that supplemental vitamin C in amounts of 250 to 500 milligrams (the DV is 60 milligrams) may lessen the symptoms. But for a person with an otherwise adequate diet, dosing with extra vitamin C has not been shown to reduce the incidence of colds. The only situation that has been scientifically proven successful is for people with a vitamin C intake that is below the DV. For them, supplemental vitamin C has been shown to reduce the number of colds. This doesn't mean that vitamin C prevents colds, but rather that an adequate intake is crucial for a healthy human immune system.

In addition to trying the zinc nasal spray and vitamin C, drink plenty of fluids and get some rest so that your immune system can do its job.

Help Heal an Injury

One summer, I tore the tendon in my kneecap. Immediately after surgery, my orthopedist put me on a rehabilitation program that included ice packs and physical therapy.

During my weeks-long break from running, cycling, and everything else that involved using that part of my body, I wondered to myself: What about a food rehab program? I figured that feeding my injury with the right foods would nourish my injured knee and help rebuild new, healthy tissue. I wanted to heal as quickly as possible. I knew that if I didn't, I might turn into one cranky (and possibly chubby) nutrition professor.

The Five Most Potent Nutritional Remedies

After my operation, I began researching how to best "feed" an injury. I wanted to know which foods were most likely to help speed the healing process. Here's a list of the five nutrition remedies, most important first, that helped me keep off the weight and get back on my feet.

1. Protein

Every day, your body makes millions of new proteins to replace the worn-out proteins in your muscles, red blood cells, connective tissues, and elsewhere. When you damage your muscles, tendons, ligaments, or joints, many of these proteins break down more rapidly than usual. Your body struggles to pump up production by forming new proteins from dietary amino acids, the building blocks of protein. To do so, however, these amino acids must be in abundant supply. If they're not, the repair process is slowed down.

You need 75 to 100 grams of protein daily (a bit more than a nonathlete) to keep up with your body's normal protein-building schedule. When you sustain an injury, you need more. As you recover, make sure that you get 80 to 110 grams of protein every day.

Also, don't skimp too much on calories. If you cut back on calories to avoid putting on extra weight, you may be delaying your recovery. If your muscles, brain, or other organs don't have enough fuel to function, they'll raid your body's protein stores, depleting those supplies even more. If you start losing weight, be wary. It could mean that you're not feeding your body enough protein to heal.

Feed your injury quality protein by incorporating eggs (or egg whites), soy, lean meats, and low-fat dairy products into your regular meals. Those foods contain all of the amino acids your body needs. Beans are also a good protein source, but combine them with a grain (such as lentil soup with cornbread) to provide a complete supply of amino acids.

2. Zinc

Your body needs zinc to manufacture healthy bone cells (called osteoblasts) and cartilage cells (called chondrocytes). If you get a stress fracture or tear some cartilage, these cells work overtime to repair the damage. Without enough zinc, your body can't make enough osteoblasts and chondrocytes to do the job.

Unfortunately, many fitness enthusiasts are already zinc deficient. If you don't eat meat or take a multivitamin/mineral supplement, you probably don't get the daily 15 milligrams that your body needs. Besides red meat, zinc-rich foods include clams and oysters. Good vegetarian sources include wheat germ, whole grain breads, and zinc-fortified breakfast cereals. Along with loading up on zinc-rich foods, you should take a multivitamin/mineral supplement that contains 100 percent of the Daily Value (DV) for zinc during your rehab.

3. Vitamin C

When you're injured, a protein called collagen forms scar tissue that glues your cells back together. Your body can't make this important substance without an adequate amount of vitamin C.

In a study done more than 30 years ago (these kinds of studies aren't done today for ethical reasons), men were fed a diet that was deficient in vitamin C (no fruits or vegetables) for several weeks. The researchers then made incisions in the men's legs and monitored the healing process. Scar formation was sparse because little collagen was present. Fortunately, the men recovered from this diet as soon as they resumed their vitamin C intake.

While this experiment was extreme, it showed the value of vitamin C for optimal healing. Aim to ingest 100 to 250 milligrams daily. Getting extra vitamin C is easy; just one orange supplies 80 milligrams. Other citrus fruits and many vegetables such as broccoli, cabbage, kale, and even potatoes are also good sources.

4. Antioxidants

When you're injured, you can blame much of the swelling and soreness you feel on things called free radicals. These highly reactive molecules damage tissue as they search for missing electrons. Antioxidants such as vitamin E and beta-carotene stop this damage by providing the electrons that free radicals need. This prevents unnecessary swelling and pain.

Eat several daily servings of fruits and vegetables such as winter squash; dark, leafy greens; kiwifruit; apples; and oranges for an array of antioxidants that includes flavonoids and carotenes. You won't find these phytochemicals in a pill, so it's time to get friendly with produce. You might also consider supplementing with 400 IU of vitamin E a day, since it's difficult to consume that amount from food alone.

5. Glucosamine

More and more physicians are telling their athlete patients about the amino acid glucosamine, which can be used as a remedy for inflammation and pain in the joints caused by overuse or injury. According to several studies, 1,500 milligrams of supplemental glucosamine may not only soothe the pain but also may actually help mend the joints. Much of the damage done to joints really involves the cartilage, and glucosamine addresses this problem by boosting the functioning of chondrocytes, the cells in your joints that make cartilage.

In addition to possibly stimulating the growth of cartilage, glucosamine also helps produce substances called glycoproteins that may speed healing in muscles, although there's no solid research yet to back up that claim.

Glucosamine is considered safe, although long-term use has not been evaluated. Consult your physician if you want to give it a try.

Calcium and Bone Breaks

While the idea is appealing and may even seem logical, taking megadoses of calcium will not heal a stress fracture any faster. The extra calcium won't rush to the fractured spot and glue the bones back together. Instead, your body will deal with the excess calcium by not absorbing it all from the digestive tract. Of the calcium that is absorbed, some is excreted in urine, while a portion gets sent to bones all over your body; the rest just passes through your system. Taking megadoses won't heal broken bones any faster but it will help strengthen them so that they don't break as easily again. Eating a high-calcium diet will do the same thing.

Stress fractures are usually caused by physical strain on your bones, not by a calcium deficiency. Some female athletes, however, who may not have regular menstrual cycles and who have low estrogen levels may develop stress fractures as a result of low calcium content in their bones. But no matter how the stress fractures develop, taking supplemental calcium is not an effective way to treat a broken bone. And you run the risk of taking in too much calcium.

At very high doses, such as 1,000 milligrams, your body's ability to absorb iron becomes impaired. Women typically have low stores of iron anyway, so too much calcium increases their risk of iron-deficiency anemia. If you ingest two or three dairy products daily, or regularly consume calcium-fortified products, you are probably already meeting your calcium needs. If you want to ensure an adequate intake every day, try a calcium supplement of no more than 500 milligrams.

Recipe Revver

Healing Seafood Stew
Serves 6

Eat this zinc-and-protein-packed stew with fresh fruit and whole grain bread to speed the healing of any injury.

- 1   tablespoon olive oil
- 2   cloves of garlic, crushed
- 1   medium onion, chopped
- 2   medium carrots, sliced
- 2   medium russet potatoes, cut into bite-size pieces
- 1   can (15 ounces) low-sodium vegetable broth
- 1   bay leaf
     Freshly ground black pepper
- 6–8 ounces fresh catfish fillet, cut into bite-size pieces
- 1   small can clams, with juice
- 1   small can (6½ ounces) oysters
- 2   ounces canned anchovies (optional)
- 2   medium tomatoes, chopped

Heat the olive oil in a large skillet over medium-high heat. Add the garlic and onion and cook, stirring frequently, for 4 minutes, or until the onions are soft. Add the carrots and the potatoes. Brown for 5 minutes. Transfer to a large soup pot and pour the broth over the vegetables. Add the bay leaf and season to taste with the black pepper. Add enough water to cover the vegetables. Bring to a boil. Simmer until the potatoes are soft but not mushy. Turn up the heat to medium-high and add the catfish. Simmer 3 to 5 minutes. Add the clams (with juice), oysters, anchovies (if using), and tomatoes. Cook for another 3 to 5 minutes. (Do not overcook; this tends to toughen clams and oysters.) Remove and discard the bay leaf.

Per serving: *223 calories, 4 g total fat, 1 g saturated fat, 23 g protein, 23 g carbohydrate, 3 g dietary fiber, 49 mg cholesterol, 960 mg sodium*

workout q&a

Q: Can eating an unhealthful diet make me more susceptible to injuries?

A: If you deprive yourself of the vitamins, minerals, protein, and other nutrients that your body needs for top performance and a speedy recovery, your eating habits will catch up with you sooner or later. Even marginal deficiencies of essential nutrients can cause significant problems when you exercise.

Nutritional deficiencies are often difficult to nip in the bud because many don't show up on routine laboratory tests. For example, early signs of depleted iron stores don't turn up unless your physician specifically tests for it. Low levels of protein, zinc, and vitamin C may not appear on regular tests either, but they may be at the root of an increased rate of injuries or illness. Since you can't always keep accurate and timely tabs on your health, you must eat for optimum health and performance every day.

While your bone fracture is healing, your best bet is to eat a healthy, well-rounded diet with adequate protein, calcium, vitamin C, and other essential nutrients. And in cases of stress fractures caused by repetitive motion and impact, time off from your exercise is crucial. You have to give the bone a break from physical stress so it can heal.

A Word about Painkillers

Many fitness enthusiasts pop painkillers as if they were candy. There's nothing wrong with using a painkiller to soothe the occasional ache or pain, but when their use becomes as automatic as your morning cup of coffee, it's time for a change in strategy.

You have a choice of five different types of painkillers: aspirin (Bayer), ibuprofen (Advil), naproxen sodium (Aleve), ketoprofen (Actron), and acetaminophen (Tylenol). All of them except for acetaminophen are designed to reduce inflammation, which is why they're called nonsteroidal anti-inflammatory drugs, or NSAIDs. They work by lowering your body's production of particular types of prostaglandins, which are hormonelike substances that are involved in numerous bodily functions, including inflammation.

But while painkillers make you feel better, they have drawbacks. Most important, if you're not careful, they can cause kidney, liver, or stomach problems. Follow these tips to stay on the safe side.

- Never pop a painkiller just before—or worse, during—a workout. Instead, listen to your body and stop exercising when it asks you to stop. Your body sends you pain signals for a reason; it's telling you to take a rest. And you should listen. If you don't, your injury will not only linger but probably get worse. When you take painkillers, you're masking pain. That may be okay if you're doing it to get to sleep at night or to get through the day at your job. But it's not okay if you're doing it so that your knee won't hurt during your next workout.
- Never take a painkiller when you are dehydrated, such as after a night of binge drinking or after a hot, sweaty race or workout. Doing so can result in kidney damage, especially in people over age 60.
- Don't make a habit out of taking painkillers. Chronic use of NSAIDs can eat away at your stomach lining and damage your kidneys. If you've been taking them every day for a month, it's time to see your doctor for a different strategy and for tests to evaluate your kidney and liver function.

Foods That Fight Pain

Try the following tips to soothe inflammation and fight pain without doing a number on your digestive tract.

Eat ginger every day. This gnarled-looking root may have natural anti-inflammatory properties that work much like ibuprofen, but without the side effects. Use a vegetable peeler to remove the outer layer, and then either grate it by hand or use a food processor to grind it. Use ½ to 1 teaspoon a day to flavor your stir-fries and other dishes; ginger tastes great added to marinades for meat and fish. You also can steep some in boiled water for a soothing tea. But don't try to eat ginger plain because it has a pungent flavor and spicy effect—you'll be drinking water for hours.

Eating Smart for...
A Day of Rehab

Use the following menu for an entire day's worth of injury-healing foods.

Breakfast
½ cup Fiber One cereal mixed with ¼ cup whole grain cereal topped with 2 teaspoons
chopped nuts

6 ounces fat-free milk

One orange

One latte made with 4 ounces fat-free milk and sprinkled with 1 tablespoon
chocolate shavings

Morning Snack
One energy bar containing 12 grams of protein (240 calories)

Lunch
1 cup fat-free cottage cheese

One tomato, chopped

3 tablespoons mixed nuts

Two medium kiwifruit

Afternoon Snack
¼ cup dried cherries and two chocolate candies

Dinner
1 cup spinach pasta tossed with ⅓ cup tomato sauce with 3 ounces clams

2 cups greens with ¼ cup whole soybeans

Calories: 1,530; Protein: 102 grams; Carbohydrate: 227 grams; Fat: 20% calories

Eat more fat. Make a special effort to ingest alpha-linolenic fat, a
heart-healthy fat in flaxseed meal, nuts, and canola oil. The omega-3
fatty acids found in fish and flaxseed may also reduce inflammation. Try
to eat a fatty fish such as salmon twice a week, and use flaxseed oil on
your salads.

Energize Your Workouts

Do you often drag yourself out of bed in the morning? Do you eye your desktop at work as a potential napping locale? Can you barely summon enough energy to make it through your workout? Are you forgetting things, struggling to concentrate, or even having trouble doing simple tasks? Is your chief complaint at the doctor's office "fatigue" or "lack of energy," so much so that your malaise is getting in the way of your work performance and home life? If your get-up-and-go has gotten up and left, it's time to take a look at your diet.

Whatever the source of your fatigue, it will affect your exercise. If you are mentally sapped, you'll opt for a nap rather than a trip to the gym. If your brain shuts down during your workout, you'll call it quits before accomplishing your goals for the day.

To boost physical energy before and during your workout, you must also build mental energy because the two go hand in hand. What you're eating (or not eating) can make the difference between crawling through your day in slow motion and feeling revved up for virtually anything.

Nine Ways to Motivate Your Body

A number of factors can conspire to make you find an excuse to not exercise. Physical hunger is the most common culprit, which is why I suggest to fitness enthusiasts that they snack on mini meals every few hours rather than eat two or three large meals a day. Other factors that mainly affect your brain's energy can cause a dip in motivation as well. Here are some food tips and strategies to keep your energy up and your motivation in motion.

1. Make Breakfast Happen

Skipping breakfast, the most important meal of the day, can leave you feeling muddleheaded both at work and during your workout. Many studies on children have shown that when they miss breakfast, they falter in reading, memory, and other cognitive skills. It appears that the brain is sensitive to short-term deficits in fuel and nutrient supply.

Going all night without food and then skipping breakfast may cause your blood sugar levels to dip, which can bring on light-headedness. And since sugar in the form of glucose is your brain's primary fuel source, it's no wonder that your memory and other thinking powers go downhill when you're running on empty.

Ready-to-eat breakfast cereal, fruit, and milk make for a great start. Or try unconventional breakfast items such as leftover pizza or a casserole. If you're in a hurry, take along a container of yogurt, a piece of fruit, and a whole grain roll, or try a ready-made pita wrap (available in your supermarket's deli section). Or throw fresh berries, low-fat ice cream, and milk in a blender, then grab a cup of this super fruit smoothie in one hand, your briefcase in the other, and go.

2. Wake Up with Water

A cold splash of water in the face has always been a reliable wake-up call, but drinking water can energize and refresh you even more. Fifty-five to 60 percent of your body is composed of water, most of it residing in your cells, where it allows for essential chemical reactions like the breakdown of carbohydrates for brain fuel. In fact, your brain is more than 70 percent water by weight, and if this percentage dips below a critical level, you'll feel listless, dull, and headachy.

Brain dehydration can easily happen even without the added stress of exercise. Dry indoor air causes fluid loss that you may not be aware of; combined with too little water intake and too many caffeinated beverages, this gradual dehydration can leave you with a brain-drain headache by late afternoon.

Keep yourself energized by starting off your morning with an 8-ounce glass of plain water before your morning coffee. Keep a bottle of water handy, drinking 1 to 2 quarts throughout the day. According to the USDA, most people in the United States drink only one-quarter of their fluid needs as plain water; they get the rest from coffee, soda, and food. For a clear head, reach for the clear stuff.

3. Snack On Raisins

Raisins (along with apples, nuts, and parsley) are a great source of the mineral boron, which plays a role in brain function, perhaps combating drowsiness. In a series of studies performed by the USDA, healthy men and women ate diets low in boron for several weeks. Another group ate the same foods but took a boron supplement. Both groups took a battery of tests that assessed brain functions such as brain wave activity and cognitive skills, including memory, attention, and manual dexterity.

Compared with those in the supplement group, the subjects on the boron-deficient diet showed slowed brain activity, indicating drowsiness. Researchers also noted deterioration in cognitive skills among the low-boron group. The USDA researchers gave the study subjects 3 to 4 milligrams of boron, a dosage equivalent to that found in about 3 ounces of raisins and 1 ounce of almonds. Toss a few raisins and nuts into your

My Food Diary

When I know that my day will be anything but serene, I start the morning with a high-energy breakfast that will fuel me with enough calories and nutrients to last until lunch. This way, I don't get light-headed or ravenous during a long lecture when I don't have time for a snack break.

I have a glass of 100-percent fruit juice and 1½ cups of nine-grain hot cereal. I stir 1 tablespoon of isolated soy protein powder into the cereal before cooking it and then add a little extra liquid. After cooking it, I stir in ¼ cup of golden raisins and 1 ounce of chopped pecans. I like to let it sit for a couple of minutes to allow the raisins and nuts to soften. Then I top it all with 6 ounces of vanilla soy milk. This breakfast gives me 582 calories, 34 grams of protein, and 68 grams of carbohydrate to start my day.

cereal and salads and keep some snack-size boxes or packets in your desk for afternoon grazing.

4. Munch On Brazil Nuts and Tuna

Brazil nuts and tuna are two of the best food sources of selenium, a mineral that not only serves as an antioxidant but also may boost mood, lift spirits, and contribute to feelings of clearheadedness. Researchers at the USDA's Human Nutrition Center in Grand Forks, North Dakota, tracked the effects of varying selenium intakes on men's mood profiles for 15 weeks. Half of the men in the study consumed 40 percent of the recommended daily selenium requirement, while the other half took in about 350 percent.

When researchers tested the moods of both groups, the high-selenium group felt more elated than depressed, more energetic than tired, more clearheaded than confused, and more confident than unsure.

But before you rush out and buy a selenium supplement, be aware that this mineral is highly toxic in large doses. Stick to no more than 400 micrograms, or five to seven times the daily requirement (which is 55 micrograms), and talk to your doctor before supplementing with that amount. Better yet, concentrate on getting selenium in your diet. In addition to tuna and nuts, other good food sources include chicken, turkey, lean beef, and whole grain bread and cereals.

5. Lighten Up at Lunch

You probably know from experience that loading up at lunch can leave you feeling sleepy in the afternoon. That's because food in your digestive tract diverts blood away from other parts of your body, leaving you with that sluggish feeling. Studies show that big meals (1,000 calories or more) at midday cause more drowsiness than lunches half that size. If you feel sleepy following even a light lunch, try adding some protein the next day.

6. Fill Up on Fiber

If you feel de-energized and hungry when your meal wears off, try adding some fiber to your fare. Pectin, a type of water-soluble fiber found in fruits such as apples and oranges, has been shown to help people feel full longer by delaying emptying of the stomach. When people swallowed a 5-gram dose of pectin (extracted from apples) with their meal, they felt full for up to 4 hours. An added benefit is that pectin also helps lower blood cholesterol levels.

7. Snack Intelligently

If you're just plain tired, eating a small snack can perk you up. Keep these snacks high in nutrient-packed, carbohydrate-rich foods and light on calories (stay under 200). If the snack is crunchy, really hot, or really cold, it will help wake up your senses. Here are some healthful examples.

- One frozen fruit bar
- 8 ounces of drinkable fruit-flavored yogurt mixed with 4 ounces of club soda
- One ready-to-eat cereal bar like Nutri-Grain tossed in the microwave for less than a minute and then spread with 1 tablespoon fat-free cream cheese
- One sorbet "sandwich" (3 tablespoons strawberry sorbet wedged between two caramel corn rice cakes)
- One small package of precut veggies with reduced-fat dip

8. Avoid a Java Jag

Drinking a cup or two of coffee improves feelings of alertness and clearheadedness and may even bolster your performance on monotonous tasks such as typing or filing. But moderate use of this pick-me-up can easily brew into a caffeine habit that may actually zap your energy and cause fatigue. People who perpetually have a cup of coffee, tea, or cola in their hands have developed a dependency. Without a steady allotment of the stimulant throughout the day, they feel tired, irritable, and even headachy (a symptom of withdrawal). In short, they're caffeine junkies.

If you view coffee or other caffeinated beverages as a life source without which you can't function, try phasing caffeine out a little at a time to regain your own natural energy. Start your "detox" by cutting one-fifth of your typical daily caffeine intake for a few weeks. You may experience fatigue or headaches for a day or two as your body goes through withdrawal. When you've adjusted to this amount, continue gradually cutting back. Once you're down to a cup or two in the morning, you can decide whether you want to eliminate caffeine altogether.

9. Ditch the Diet

According to research, people who cut calories to slim down perform poorly on tests of memory and mental processing. One study compared the mental performances of people on weight-reducing diets to the performances of those who weren't dieting. The researchers likened the slowed mental performance seen in dieters to being intoxicated by alcohol.

While some researchers argue that poor mental performance stems from an inadequate flow of energy to the brain, the researchers who did the study theorize that the results of the study reflect dieters' feelings of anxiety. When dieting, most people start obsessing over the foods that they are trying not to eat as well as worrying about the success of their dieting efforts. This type of distraction affects mental processing capacity. The effects were more serious in dieters who weren't losing weight than in those who were, supporting the theory that anxiety may play a role in undermining mental performance.

If you're limiting your calories to lose weight, avoid radical dieting, which is sure to leave you feeling drained. The best route to weight loss is to boost your activity level to burn more calories while simultaneously making small adjustments to your eating habits. You have better things to do than worry about your next meal.

The Brain's Role in Fitness Fatigue

Feeling bushed at the end of a hard workout is perfectly normal. In fact, it's inevitable; you're not a machine, and fatigue is your body's way of telling you that enough is enough. But if you've been extra tired lately after your usual workouts, there might be more to it than physical exhaustion. You could be experiencing brain fatigue.

Researchers have long pondered the origin of exercise fatigue, and they now agree that several factors contribute to it, including spent stores of muscle glycogen, overuse of specific muscle groups through repeated contractions, and lactic acid buildup. These are what exercise physiologists call peripheral fatigue mechanisms; they originate in the muscles themselves.

Research shows, however, that exercise fatigue is also caused by mechanisms in the brain. Specifically, scientists look at neurotransmitters—brain chemicals responsible for mood and alertness, among other things. They believe that levels of the neurotransmitter serotonin rise during exercise and cause fatigue.

This brain theory, or central fatigue hypothesis of exercise exhaustion, was developed by Eric Newsholme, Ph.D., a biochemist at Oxford University in England. When you exercise for long periods, your muscles become drained of glycogen, which is the form that carbohydrates take when stored in your muscle tissue. When glycogen stores run low, fatty acids released from fat cells become a primary energy source.

Fatty acids require a special carrier to take them through your bloodstream. The problem is that another substance called tryptophan (an amino acid that the brain converts to serotonin) rides this same carrier. What happens is that during endurance exercise, increasing numbers of fatty acids bump tryptophan off its carrier. The free-floating tryptophan enters your brain, where it converts to serotonin. As a result, serotonin levels increase and you feel like bagging your workout.

This fatty acid–tryptophan–serotonin chain of events isn't the only mechanism responsible for brain fatigue. There's a second biochemical interaction that brings on fatigue. It involves substances called branched-chain amino acids (BCAAs) that compete with tryptophan for entry into your brain.

During a long bout of exercise, such as a marathon or century bike ride, your muscles use BCAAs for fuel. This lowers the amount of circu-

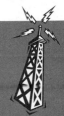

Nutrition News Flash

If you've been diagnosed with chronic fatigue syndrome, consider taking a B-complex vitamin. A study published in the *Journal of the Royal Society of Medicine* found that people with chronic fatigue syndrome are usually deficient in the B vitamins pyridoxine, riboflavin, and thiamin. More research is needed to find out if a deficiency causes the condition, or if people with chronic fatigue syndrome somehow have trouble absorbing or processing these vitamins. Either way, a B-complex multivitamin can't hurt.

Find a B-complex vitamin that provides 100 to 200 percent of the Daily Value.

Eating Smart for...
High Energy

Try the following menu to perk up your energy levels.

Breakfast
> One whole wheat pita spread with 2 tablespoons peanut butter and stuffed with half of a sliced banana
> 8 ounces grapefruit juice

Morning Snack
> 1-ounce mozzarella cheese stick
> Four dried apricot halves

Lunch
> 1 cup black-bean soup
> 1 cup fruit salad
> 8 ounces 1% milk or soy milk

Afternoon Snack
> ½ cup trail mix (dried mango, raisins, walnuts) sprinkled over 1 cup vanilla yogurt

Dinner
> 3 ounces grilled fish
> ¾ cup polenta
> 1 cup green beans and 1 medium sliced tomato drizzled with 1 tablespoon olive oil and 2 tablespoons basil

Evening Snack
> One oatmeal cookie spread with 3 tablespoons frozen yogurt

Calories: 2,250; Protein: 94 grams; Carbohydrate: 323 grams; Fat: 29% calories

lating BCAAs, which means that more tryptophan can get into your brain because it doesn't have to compete with as many BCAAs to do so. As a result, more serotonin is produced and fatigue sets in. Theoretically, if you could maintain higher levels of BCAAs in your bloodstream during exercise, more BCAAs and less tryptophan would get into your brain, and this would help fight fatigue.

Food for Thought

The key to fighting brain fatigue during exercise is to prevent tryptophan from getting into your brain in the first place. Certain foods, particularly those rich in carbohydrate, can help accomplish this.

When you take in carbohydrate just before or during exercise, your muscles use the carbohydrate as fuel and send a signal to your fat cells to slow the release of fatty acids. This decreases the amount of tryptophan going to your brain.

To examine the carbohydrate-brain connection, Mark Davis, Ph.D., an exercise physiologist at the University of South Carolina in Columbia, put trained cyclists to the test. Two groups of cyclists were asked to pedal on stationary bikes at two-thirds of their maximum effort until exhaustion. While cycling, they drank 8 ounces of fluid every 30 minutes. The first group drank a placebo beverage that contained no carbohydrate, while the second group drank a sports drink loaded with carbohydrate.

The cyclists who drank the placebo stopped pedaling after about 3 hours. Those who ingested the carbohydrate lasted a full 45 minutes longer. Researchers also discovered that the levels of free fatty acids and tryptophan climbed to more than 500 percent of normal in the placebo group and were highest at the time of exhaustion. Those who consumed the carbohydrate had far lower levels of both.

"The carbohydrate beverages clearly boosted performance in these cyclists," says Dr. Davis. "And while some of the improvement may be from increased fuel for the muscles, our results show that carbohydrate also plays a role in delaying fatigue through central mechanisms." In other words, carbohydrate holds down levels of fatty acids and tryptophan.

The Chain Gang

The theory that you can take a dose of BCAAs while exercising so that less tryptophan reaches the brain for serotonin production sounds plausible, but studies have been inconclusive. According to Dr. Davis, the quantity of BCAAs needed to lessen the amount of tryptophan entering the brain would be poorly tolerated and perhaps even dangerous. BCAA beverages taste awful, and they slow fluid absorption, which increases the risk of dehydration. They also tend to cause cramping and gastrointestinal upset. And worse, heavy doses could possibly bring about toxic levels of ammonia in your body.

Yet sports drinks containing BCAAs have already hit the market. While testimonials from endurance athletes suggest that these beverages do ward off fatigue, the amount of BCAAs in these products—less than 1 gram per serving—is small and would have negligible effects. Until more is learned about BCAAs and fatigue, avoid taking excessive amounts of supplements containing these amino acids.

Instead of loading up on BCAAs to fight brain fatigue, try the following strategies before and during your workouts and races.

- Eat high-carbohydrate foods such as cereal, bread, low-fat muffins, or fruit 2 to 3 hours before a long workout. The carbohydrate will be released into your bloodstream during your workout, where it will serve as fuel for exercising muscles and help stave off brain fatigue.
- Avoid fasting. Skipping a meal shortly before a workout or race not only can leave you short on fuel but also can lead to brain fatigue. Glycogen stores become depleted, so your body compensates by increasing the circulation of fatty acids for fuel. As fatty acid levels go up, so does your level of tryptophan and your level of fatigue.
- Keep away from high-fat foods before your workouts. Doughnuts, fatty meats, or full-fat dairy products may cause early fatigue by increasing the levels of circulating fatty acids.
- During a long exercise session, eat carbohydrate foods that have a high glycemic index (a measure of how quickly a carbohydrate food is processed, releasing sugar into the bloodstream). These foods are exactly what you need to fuel your muscles and keep fatty acid levels from climbing. Good choices include sports drinks, raisins, bread, potatoes, and cookies sweetened with molasses.
- Get adequate rest. Early fatigue during workouts or races may be a sign that you're not getting adequate rest and recovery. If you play hard on a daily basis, be sure to get plenty of sleep at night. And once a week or so, schedule a day for rest or for light cross-training to give your muscles—and mind—a break from hard training.

chapter sixteen

Enhance Your Endurance

Endurance means different things to different people. Whether you define it as backpacking through wine country, cycling through Germany, finishing a triathlon, or simply playing hard longer, you need to pay careful attention to what you eat and drink. Without the right fuel, your body will run out of gas. Just as important, the right performance diet will ensure that your endurance exercise improves your health and doesn't detract from it.

There is a limit to the health benefits of continuous, high-intensity exercise. That limit seems to be 2 to 4 hours, depending on the type of exercise. Once you go past that point, the extra oxygen you breathe, the extra use of your muscles, and the general wear and tear on your body starts to lower your immunity and increase inflammation. It may also increase your risk of chronic disease by allowing free radicals to damage your cells, making them more prone to attack by carcinogens and other threats.

The right foods and beverages can halt this destructive process, helping you to exercise longer and better.

Don't Bonk

Your muscles run on a type of stored energy called glycogen, which is made from the carbohydrate that you consume in your diet. As you exercise, your body drains stored carbohydrate from your muscles. Unless you replenish those stores, your body will run out of this fuel after about 90 minutes. As your muscles begin to pull sugar out of your bloodstream as a backup, your blood sugar plummets, setting off a chain of reactions in your brain that make you feel dead tired.

Cyclists call this sensation bonking; runners call it hitting the wall. And that's pretty much what it feels like. If you've ever seen a pale-faced cyclist or runner stumbling around and asking others for food, you know that bonking is something that you don't want to experience.

Studies show that consuming some form of carbohydrate as little as a half-hour into your workout can help you exercise longer and more intensely without hitting the wall. That's because carbohydrate keeps your blood sugar levels steady, which in turn helps your muscles access more fuel. As an added benefit, regular carbohydrate consumption also keeps your immunity high and may even keep your brain operating on all four cylinders (or lobes).

For best results, consume 30 to 60 grams of carbohydrate for every hour of exercise. That comes to 120 to 240 calories per hour. The key here is to fuel up while you're exercising. If you wait until after an hour has gone by, it's too late. You want to keep a steady supply of carbohydrate entering your bloodstream, so try to consume 60 to 120 calories every half-hour. The exact right amount depends on your body size and exercise intensity, and the best way to consume these calories depends on you and your exercise pursuits. Experiment with sports drinks, carbohydrate-rich energy bars, dried fruit, bananas, and energy gels. You'll find that some types of food work better for you than others.

You also want to eat plenty of carbohydrate when you're not exercising, to keep your muscles well-stocked with fuel. The optimal training diet includes 60 percent of your calories from carbohydrate, 25 percent from fat, and 15 percent from protein. For the average 2,800-calorie-per-day diet, this breaks down to 420 grams of carbohydrate, 77 grams of fat, and 105 grams of protein. That will give you plenty of carbohydrate to replenish spent glycogen stores. You'll also get lots of protein for repairing your hard-working muscles and for keeping your immune system strong.

Fitting In Fat

Some endurance athletes get carried away with carbohydrate. Instead of 60 poroont, thoy oat olooor to 00 pcrocnt of their calories from carbohydrate. But more isn't necessarily better; in fact, it's worse. Your body needs protein and fat, too.

Fat may bc morc important for endurance performance than was once thought. In one study, exercise physiologists Ted Zderic and Ed Coyle from the University of Texas at Austin fed endurance cyclists varying amounts of fat. The experiment tested three different diets: very high carbohydrate and very low fat (88 percent and 2 percent of calories, respectively); high carbohydrate and low fat (68 percent and 21 percent of calories, respectively); and moderate carbohydrate and high fat (57 percent and 32 percent of calories, respectively).

The cyclists spent 5 days on each diet and did a 2-hour ride every day. While on the first diet, the cyclists had glycogen stores that were packed to the max, but their levels of muscle fat were scanty. The second diet supplied enough fat to give the cyclists the same amount of muscle fat as the third, high-fat diet. The second diet also packed the cyclists' glycogen stores almost to capacity.

Muscle fat is very important to endurance. Referred to as intra-muscular triglyceride, this stored fat is a vital

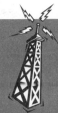

Nutrition News Flash

According to research from exercise physiologists Donovan Fogt and John Ivy, Ph.D., at the University of Texas at Austin, a combination of carbohydrate and protein may refuel your muscles faster than carbohydrate alone.

In the study, endurance cyclists rode for 2 hours to deplete their muscle glycogen stores. Immediately following the rides and again 2 hours later, the cyclists drank 12 ounces of a carbohydrate-and-protein beverage (53 grams of carbohydrate and 14 grams of protein) or a sports drink (20 grams of carbohydrate). Those who drank the carbohydrate-and-protein beverage had a 128 percent greater restocking of glycogen compared with those who had the carbohydrate-only sports drink.

Some good combinations include a tuna sandwich on whole grain bread along with a peach, or an energy bar containing 15 grams of protein and 8 ounces of high-carbohydrate sports drink such as Gatorade Torq.

source of fuel during exercise, supplying more than 60 percent of the total fat used to power your body. Skimping on fat in the diet may leave you short on muscle fuel, so enjoy healthy fats such as nuts, avocado, and fatty fish.

Staying Healthy for the Long Haul

If you've ever come down with a bad cold after running a marathon or finishing another long-distance event, you're not alone; 25 percent of distance runners report falling ill after an endurance event such as a marathon. Studies show that the immune system is suppressed for up to 72 hours after high-effort endurance exercise, creating an open window for invading bacteria and viruses. One theory as to the cause is that your immune system begins repairing the minor damage inflicted on your muscles and tendons and essentially gets distracted from fighting off invading germs. Here are some tips to keep your immune system running strong.

Focus on carbohydrate. Research done by David C. Nieman, Ph.D., professor of health and exercise science at Appalachian State University in Boone, North Carolina, suggests that quaffing a sports drink during an endurance event may bolster your immune system.

Fifty marathon runners were given either sports drink or a placebo beverage to drink during a race at a rate of 1 liter per hour of running. This amounts to 60 grams of carbohydrate (or 240 calories) per hour. Dr. Nieman took blood samples from the runners before, immediately after, and 1½ hours after the marathon and analyzed them for immune system function and strength. The runners who drank the sports drink showed improved measures of certain specialized immune cells, suggesting a better defense against illness.

Eat more vegetables. If you're the type of person who plays hard almost every day, you need to eat lots of vegetables. Nutrients such as carotenoids (substances that your body converts to vitamin A) and vitamins C and E are found abundantly in produce. These nutrients neutralize the free radicals created during exercise. Citrus fruits, carrots, green, leafy vegetables, and other types of fruits and vegetables are loaded with these protective substances. Eat as many different fruits and vegetables as you can—eight or more servings each day.

Check out the fish department. Fish contains important fats that fight inflammation and boost immunity. Aim for two servings a week of fatty cold-water fish such as salmon or mackerel.

Pop some vitamin C. Several studies done on South African ultramarathon runners show that taking 600 milligrams of vitamin C every day for 3 weeks after the endurance effort may lower the risk of catching a cold.

Avoid sick people. After a long endurance effort, try to minimize your exposure to people with colds or flu. While you can't ignore your own runny-nosed children, you can avoid enclosed public places such as movie theaters and airline flights.

Wash up. Wash your hands before eating or touching your face to prevent transmitting any potentially harmful invaders.

Maintaining Brain Power

To go that extra mile, your brain needs to be just as committed as your body. Fuel up with the wrong foods, and the neurotransmitters in your brain will tell your body to go on strike. Your muscles will be perfectly stocked with fuel, but your brain will say, "I'm tired, let's quit." This happens because levels of the brain chemical serotonin rise during exercise, eventually causing fatigue.

If you can keep your serotonin levels from spiking, you'll keep your brain (and body) energized. Eating a high-carbohydrate snack just before or during exercise will do the trick. This prevents the release of free fatty acids, which decreases the production of serotonin in your brain. In addition to carbohydrate, some researchers think that ingesting a substance called branched-chain amino acids (BCAAs) during exercise may also prevent brain fatigue. Although the theory sounds plausible, studies have been inconclusive, so stay away from the stuff.

The Right Recovery

After a grueling 4-hour bike ride, all-day hike, or long run, you may want to take a shower and go to sleep. Or you may want to celebrate your effort with a few beers.

Both of those choices will make any amount of exercise you plan to do the next day nearly impossible. If you exercise for long durations on a

Eating Smart for...
Enhancing Endurance

Fuel up with the following meals to get the right amount of carbohydrate, protein, and fat in your diet.

Breakfast
1½ cups of nine-grain cereal topped with 1 teaspoon chopped walnuts, 1 tablespoon honey, and 2 tablespoons dried cherries
One slice whole grain bread spread with 1 tablespoon peanut butter
1 cup blueberries with 6 ounces 1% milk

Lunch
1 cup bean salad made with 2 tablespoons olive oil and vinegar dressing
One 3-inch square of cornbread spread with 2 tablespoons apple butter
1 cup fruit salad (strawberries, cantaloupe, grapes)
8 ounces vanilla soy milk

Afternoon Snack
½ cup soy nuts with dried papaya and pineapple
8 ounces mango juice

Dinner
4 ounces grilled tuna over 1 cup curried rice mixed with 2 tablespoons pine nuts
2 cups spring mix salad tossed with half a red bell pepper, 1 ounce goat cheese, and 2 tablespoons raspberry vinaigrette dressing
1 cup apple cobbler made with oats, brown sugar, and walnut topping

Calories: 2,335; Protein: 92 grams; Carbohydrate: 370 grams; Fat: 23% calories

regular basis, or if you are planning to do a multiday endurance event such as an eco-challenge, you need to pay just as much attention to what you eat after exercise as you do before and during. If you don't, no amount of eating before and during exercise will fuel your efforts the next time you work out.

After a long bout of exercise, you need to consume calories and fluids immediately. Your muscles are most receptive to carbohydrate replenishment during the first hour after exercise. You need only 100 to 400 calories. Drinking two glasses of a caloric beverage such as a sports drink, milk, or orange juice immediately after your exercise session will give you the calories you need.

After an endurance effort, you need more than one meal. Follow those first 100 to 400 calories by eating high-carbohydrate foods along with some protein every 2 to 4 hours. Good choices include sandwiches, bean burritos, vegetables tossed with pasta and cheese, cottage cheese with fruit, baked potatoes topped with chili, and rice with tofu or chicken. Replace your fluids as well by drinking frequently.

Following a long workout, consume 2,400 calories in the next 24 hours, and pace yourself at about 50 grams of carbohydrate every 2 hours, on average.

Build
Muscle

When I attend conferences where scientists spout off their latest findings on muscle building, I often hear people snickering in the back of the room, "Come *o-o-on*, buddy; we've known that for years. Tell us something we don't already know."

Indeed, among the various types of fitness enthusiasts, bodybuilders seem to be the most widely read. Scientists usually study supplements and eating habits based on what bodybuilders are already doing, which is why research always seems to be behind the times.

That's also why many bodybuilders won't wait for scientists to test fad diets and supplements to see if they work or, more important, to see if they are safe. Instead, many bodybuilders treat themselves like laboratory rats, trying anything and everything in the pursuit of big muscles.

There's a big problem with self-experimentation, however: It could kill you.

Even though it can sometimes take years for science to catch up with and study the products being sold at vitamin and health food stores, it's research that is needed. I don't want to try any fad until someone has determined how it will affect my health. And that's why hard-core bodybuilders may find this chapter somewhat conservative. I won't recom-

mend anything that hasn't been proven safe. On the other hand, everything in this chapter is proven to build muscle.

Building muscle is a very simple science. To build muscle, you must
synthesize more protein than your body breaks down. Doing so requires
a combination of smart weight lifting and smart eating.

Timing

Working out on an empty stomach can be detrimental to muscle
growth for two reasons. First, your muscles need fuel to grow. Second, if
you feel tired, you won't be able to lift as much weight.

When it comes to weight lifting, eating before your workout may be
more important than eating after. In one study, people consumed a beverage with 6 grams of essential amino acids and 35 grams of carbohydrate just before or just after weight training. Their muscles responded
better when they drank the beverage before the exercise.

Those who work out on an empty stomach usually do so first thing in
the morning. Consuming 6 grams of protein and 35 grams of carbohydrate is easy if you know what you're doing. You need to take in only 164
calories; here are a few tasty ideas.

- Eat a small energy bar that contains both protein and carbohydrate.
- Swallow a smoothie made with strawberries, banana, nonfat yo-
  gurt, and a carton of pasteurized liquid egg substitute.
- Drink two glasses of fat-free milk.
- Eat a container of fruit-flavored yogurt.

In the Gym

During the first few months of a weight-lifting program, most people
get results quickly and easily. Your muscles get hard and start to grow,
and it seems like every time you go to the gym, you're able to lift heavier
weights. The fat melts away. Then you hit a plateau. Once your progress
starts to drop off, try the following tips.

Slow down. In their zeal to heft more weight, many people use poor
lifting form. Besides not efficiently challenging your muscles, poor form

workout q&a

Q: I have been doing a combination of 200 crunches and situps every day, but my stomach still doesn't have that "six-pack" look. What am I doing wrong?

A: You may think that the more you exercise your abs, the better they'll look, but it's not possible to rid your midriff of body fat with situps or crunches, no matter how many you do. Overall fitness—a combination of cardiovascular fitness and muscle strength—is what you need to focus on. Staying in good condition helps keep your body fat levels low, giving your entire frame a leaner, more toned look. Regular aerobic workouts of brisk walking, kickboxing, jogging, or cycling three or four times a week, along with strength training, will help you achieve your fitness goals.

In addition to your regular abdominal exercises, add side stomach crunches to work your oblique muscles (found on the sides of your torso). Lying on your back with your knees bent, lift your upper body off the ground while twisting to bring your right shoulder toward your left knee. Lower yourself back to the floor. Lift your upper body again, this time bringing your left shoulder toward your right knee. Repeat 15 to 30 times on each side.

can also result in an injury. Slow down, do fewer reps, and do them right. And *never* cheat by bouncing the lifting bar off your chest.

Stop talking so much. Many people spend hours at the gym, but spend very little of that time actually lifting weights. Rather, it's spent chatting with the person on the stair-stepper or rambling on about last night's game. Rest breaks can sometimes stretch beyond 3 minutes, and your workout suffers. Set a countdown timer on your watch to beep 1½ minutes after every set. As soon as it sounds, start lifting, no matter how juicy your current conversation.

Mix it up. Once your body adapts to a particular motion, it doesn't have to work as hard to accomplish the task. Mix up your weight-lifting moves. For example, instead of always bench-pressing to work your chest, try chest flies, pushups, and chinups. Instead of always doing biceps curls, try preacher curls or concentration curls. Instead of always doing dips for your triceps, try kickbacks and skull crushers.

Change your sets. Alternate between two sets of 15 reps, three sets of 8 reps, and a drop set of 8 hard reps and then an immediate set of 15 reps with a lighter weight.

Work smaller muscle groups. You probably do efficient lifting exercises that work large muscle groups in your chest, back, arms, and legs. But your smaller individual muscles are also important. Though those large muscle groups will grow fast and make you look muscular, the smaller ones will help you continue working out. Pay special attention to the rotator cuff muscles in your shoulders, which will help you bench-press more weight without injury.

Rest. When it comes to weight lifting, more isn't necessarily better. Your muscles do most of their growing while you are resting, not while you are lifting. Various studies have found that working the same muscle without a 48-hour break between sessions is actually counterproductive. Never lift more often than every other day for the same muscle groups. And consider taking a few days off. Surprisingly, fewer sessions may net you bigger results.

In the Kitchen

Muscles need fuel to grow. If you don't eat, all of the weight lifting in the world won't make your muscles larger. You need 2,500 extra calories to build 1 pound of muscle. And you burn 300 to 500 calories during every hour that you lift weights, so you need to eat a lot. Here are some pointers on what types of food should make up the majority of those calories.

Protein

With heavy training, you need extra protein in your diet. Studies show that weight lifting boosts protein needs an estimated 50 percent or more above the Daily Value (DV).

Your protein requirement is based on your body weight. The recommended amount for protein is 0.36 gram per pound of body weight—about 65 grams for a person who weighs 180 pounds. But the extra 50 percent bumps the requirement up to about 100 grams daily for the same athlete. Your body uses the extra protein for building and repairing muscle tissue, and also burns small amounts for fuel. Most people easily meet their increased protein needs simply by eating foods such as fish, lean meats, soy, eggs, beans, and dairy products.

A 3-ounce serving of fish or lean meat (the size of a deck of cards) alone has 21 grams of protein. But being a musclehead doesn't necessarily mean that you have to be a meathead. With some careful planning, even vegetarians can get enough protein in their diets to beef up.

Soy, eggs, or milk proteins are great fuel sources that our bodies use very efficiently. Many bodybuilders take protein supplements, but they are paying more than they need to. You get virtually the same amount of protein from a tofu stir-fry or a container of yogurt as you do from a supplement. On the other hand, supplements are convenient if your hectic schedule prevents you from fixing real meals. Protein powder is easily added to blender drinks, soups, or other foods. Most supplements provide 15 to 30 grams of protein per serving.

One of the problems with supplements is that you can easily consume more protein than your body needs, and for some people this may be risky. Your kidneys process the extra protein your body doesn't need, and then your body burns it as fuel or converts it to fat and stores it for later use. People with kidney disease should avoid extra protein. If you have a family history of kidney disease, see your physician before adding any type of protein supplements to your diet.

Some weight lifters argue that certain sources of protein are better than others. Supplement manufacturers would like you to believe this, too, but research simply doesn't back up this claim. Whey protein, egg protein, and soy protein all go to the same place.

What is important is that you get plenty of essential amino acids, which is easy. As long as you stick with complete protein sources such as eggs, dairy, and soy, you'll consume all the essential amino acids you need.

Carbohydrate

Too many bodybuilders put all of the emphasis on protein, but carbohydrate is just as important for a number of reasons. You can use one-

Recipe Revver

Power Burrito
Makes 1

One of these easy-to-fix burritos and some fresh fruit makes a great prelifting meal. The filling can be stored for up to 2 weeks in the refrigerator and can also be used in casseroles and as a dip for fresh vegetables.

¾ cup refried black beans
1 tablespoon soy powder
¼ teaspoon red-pepper flakes
2 tablespoons green salsa
½ cup brown rice
2 tablespoons reduced-fat Monterey Jack cheese
1 spinach or whole wheat tortilla

Combine the beans, soy powder, pepper flakes, salsa, rice, and cheese. Spoon the mixture into the tortilla and roll closed. Microwave on high for 1 minute or until heated through.

Per burrito: *575 calories, 52 g protein, 89 g carbohydrate, 9 g total fat, 4 g saturated fat, 20 mg cholesterol, 8 g dietary fiber, 450 mg sodium*

quarter to one-half of the glycogen stores in your muscles, depending on how intensely you lift and the number of sets you perform. The only way you can replace that glycogen is by eating carbohydrate. Without it, you'll feel like a 200-pound weakling. And if you burn all of your stored carbohydrate during a session of lifting, your body starts eating up protein, which makes your muscles smaller, not bigger.

More encouraging is the fact that loading up with carbohydrate before hitting the gym may help you recover fast and build bigger muscles during the hours following your workout. Research shows that carbohydrate ingestion may stimulate the hormone insulin, which can shuttle those amino acids to your muscles. Combining carbohydrate with protein as a snack before you lift weights is probably the most effective way to build bigger muscles.

Shoot for 15 to 20 servings of carbohydrate a day. The average bowl

Eating Smart for...
Muscle Building

Try the following menu for building bigger muscles.

Breakfast
Fruit smoothie (6 ounces pasteurized liquid egg substitute, 4 ounces vanilla soy milk,
1 cup frozen blueberries, 4 ounces cranberry juice, crushed ice)
One whole wheat English muffin spread with 1 teaspoon trans-free margarine and
1 tablespoon jam

Lunch
One tuna sandwich (two slices whole wheat bread, 3 ounces tuna, 2 teaspoons reduced-
fat mayonnaise, lettuce, two tomato slices)
½ cup baked corn chips
1 cup fruit salad (pineapple, peaches, kiwifruit)

Afternoon Snack
Half of an energy bar
16 ounces sports drink

Dinner
1½ cups bean-and-turkey chili
1 cup brown rice
1 cup red and green bell pepper slices dipped in 2 tablespoons reduced-fat dressing
Two oatmeal cookies

Calories: 2,082; Protein: 104 grams; Carbohydrate: 332 grams; Fat: 18% calories

of Shredded Wheat cereal topped with a banana counts as five servings. Two sandwiches (made with four slices of bread) make four more. A pasta salad and baked potato for dinner offer nine more servings. Snacking on bagels and muffins brings you up to 20.

Creatine
Weight lifting depends on creatine phosphate for fuel, and you can burn almost all of your stores during a session. If you supplement with 20 to 25 grams of creatine for 5 to 7 days, you can boost your levels by 20 to 30 per-

cent. As a result, you'll be able to lift a heavier weight more times. Creatine supplementation does help build muscle size; in one study, weight lifters took creatine for 6 weeks and experienced significant gains in lean tissue.

Other studies, however, show minimal (if any) improvement in muscle-mass gains, and few studies have looked at the supplement's long-term safety, especially in adolescents. But the biggest problem with creatine is that the effects don't last. Once you stop taking it, the performance benefits disappear. And researchers don't know what happens to your body's ability to make its own supply of creatine if you stay on the supplements for an extended period of time.

Vitamins

Fit people, including bodybuilders, have a higher demand for many vitamins, minerals, and other nutrients, so it's a good idea to take a daily multivitamin/mineral supplement and to pump up your consumption of fruits, vegetables, and whole grains.

You may wonder whether taking a multivitamin just before a workout boosts the effectiveness of the supplement. It doesn't. Your muscles do need nutrients like thiamin and niacin to be able to use carbohydrate and fat as fuel for driving muscle contraction and movement. But these nutrients are already available for quick use inside your muscle cells.

And it takes 20 minutes to several hours for the vitamins and minerals in a pill to be distributed throughout your body. Even if there were an exercise benefit to topping off your nutrient levels, any such charge probably wouldn't kick in until after your workout was over.

Finally, most multivitamin/mineral supplements are best absorbed with food. Get in the habit of taking your capsule with your morning meal rather than waiting until later, when your routine might be ruined.

chapter eighteen

Increase Your Speed

Nutrition scientists used to lavish all of their research attention on endurance athletes. And that made sense. When you run, cycle, swim, or walk for a long period of time, you eventually use up all of the stored fuel in your muscles, which makes you feel tired. Many nutrition researchers didn't spend any time studying sprinters and other athletes driven by speed because they didn't think nutrition made much of a difference.

Because sprinters run or cycle for just a brief period of time, it doesn't seem logical that they could run out of fuel like endurance athletes, but they can and they do. And researchers are only beginning to unravel the best eating strategies for these types of exercise pursuits.

Gauging Energy Drain

High-intensity exercise burns the stored glycogen in your muscles at a very high rate, even if it lasts only the few seconds it takes you to run from third base to home plate. Once you stop your effort, your body stops burning fuel. One short sprint may drain your glycogen fuel tanks by only 5 percent or so, but multiple short bursts of activity, such as in a game of football or baseball, can drain those tanks to empty.

And your body doesn't drain fuel from your muscle fibers at the same rate. Even though you may have plenty of fuel left in your "slow-twitch" fibers, your body isn't necessarily using it, preferring instead to suck all the energy it can from your "fast-twitch" fibers. As a result, your fast-twitch fibers run out of fuel and you slow down.

The Right Fuel for the Short Sprint

Besides helping you stock more fuel in your muscles, the right diet will increase your body's ability to handle the lactic acid that accumulates. It also will interact with various neurotransmitters in your brain, helping you feel less fatigued.

Fueling up with a high-carbohydrate diet is the key to getting the nutrients you need for increasing speed. Many studies show that sprinters perform better on a high-carbohydrate diet; the time it takes for them to feel exhaustion is increased by 18 to 50 percent. Studies also show that the people who take part in speed sports tend to eat a low-carbohydrate diet of only 36 to 53 percent of total calories, compared to the recommended 55 to 65 percent that you need to perform at your best. That's probably because many sprinters falsely believe that they must eat lots of protein to create the large muscles needed for the job.

During competitions where multiple sprinting efforts are needed, such as in a game of soccer or baseball, guzzle some sports drink while you're standing on the sidelines. Sipping a drink that contains carbohydrate between events or efforts can help keep your muscles fueled.

Caffeine

Studies have shown that the amount of caffeine contained in about 2 cups of coffee, consumed about 1 hour before exercise, can help boost your endurance, possibly by encouraging your body to burn more fat as a fuel, thus conserving valuable glycogen. This made researchers from the University of Melbourne in Australia wonder whether caffeine might also give a boost to shorter efforts such as sprint rowing.

Competitive oarswomen were given either one of two doses of caffeine (one equivalent to 4 cups of coffee, the other equivalent to 6 cups) or a placebo 1 hour before a timed 2,000-meter rowing event. The higher

Eating Smart for...
Speed

Follow this menu to get the right proportion of carbohydrate, protein, and fat.

Breakfast
Two poached eggs on one whole grain English muffin

1 cup fruit salad (peaches, mango, oranges) topped with ½ cup yogurt

Lunch
One chicken burrito (rice, beans, 3 ounces chicken, 1 ounce Cheddar cheese wrapped in one whole wheat tortilla)

⅓ cup each celery, jicama, and radishes dipped in 2 tablespoons salsa-ranch dressing

One oatmeal cookie

8 ounces fat-free milk

Afternoon Snack
Two dried pear halves

8 ounces sports drink

Dinner
3 ounces grilled shrimp with ¾ cup roasted red and green bell peppers over ¾ cup saffron rice

2 cups spinach salad with ½ cup chopped tomato and 1 tablespoon poppy seed dressing

½ cup pineapple sorbet drizzled with 1 tablespoon chocolate syrup

Calories: 2,200; Protein: 90 grams; Carbohydrate: 317 grams; Fat: 26% calories

dose of caffeine improved sprint times by about 1½ seconds, with most of that improvement occurring during the first 500 meters of the race. The researchers note that caffeine stimulates the adrenal glands, which revs up your body's fight-or-flight response. But they also note that at this high dosage, some of the rowers tested over the International Olympic Committee's legal limit for caffeine.

If you enjoy coffee or another caffeinated beverage before training or racing, you may get off to a faster start. But be aware that 4 to 6 cups of coffee may cause nervousness, increased fluid losses through urine, and an irregular heartbeat. It also increases your heart and breathing rates.

Ribose

Inside every cell in your body, the simple sugar ribose interacts with a high-energy molecule called adenosine triphosphate (ATP), which you need for most of the chemical reactions that take place in your body. Since your body manufactures its own ribose, no one considered it a factor in exercise performance.

Researchers from Eastern Michigan University in Ypsilanti speculated that supplements could boost ribose levels inside your cells, which in turn would increase your pool of ATP. The result would be greater speed and power.

To test this theory, the researchers gave cyclists either four 8-gram doses of ribose or a placebo over a 36-hour period. The cyclists then performed six 10-second sprints on stationary bikes while the researchers measured peak power output.

Ribose supplementation did indeed boost peak power in four of the six sprint efforts. The researchers agree that more studies need to be done, but they say that ribose supplementation shows promise as a speed-enhancing aid.

It's too early to recommend spending money on ribose supplements, but these products are already on the market, and plenty of people will try them out. Since ribose is a simple sugar, it probably doesn't pose adverse health effects beyond possible weight gain from the extra calories.

chapter nineteen

Sharpen Your Golf Game

I know many people (especially people who don't play golf) who consider golf more of a hobby than a sport. Because they don't see a lot of sweating going on, they assume that there must not be any exercise going on, either.

But those of us who carry our own clubs and leave the carts behind know better. And people who play speed golf get even more of a workout.

Whether you walk or run from green to green, a full game of golf will keep you on the links for hours. During those hours, you burn calories, sweat out fluids, test your stamina, and concentrate more than you do during a typical day at work. If you walk rather than ride in a cart, you may cover 4 to 5 miles, depending on the layout of the course. You'll burn 500 or more calories by the end of the game. Lugging your own clubs burns an additional 100 to 150 calories. And swinging the club gives your back, hips, butt, and thighs a good workout.

Add all this exercise together, and you're in need of proper performance nutrition. Unfortunately, many golfers think that the only performance food they need on the course is a six-pack of beer.

A day spent on the golf course requires you to be vigilant about several things: staying well-hydrated, eating every 2 to 4 hours to maintain blood sugar levels, and avoiding foods and beverages that will interfere with your hand-eye coordination and concentration. Here's a look at each.

Staying Hydrated on the Links

You can lose a liter or more of sweat in an hour of golfing. If you're lugging clubs, your sweat loss can be even greater. And if you don't replenish lost sweat, your performance will lag. Light-headedness, fatigue, and nausea are tell-tale signs of dehydration. Don't wait until you feel thirsty; thirst typically lags behind true dehydration, signaling you to drink up long after you get stuck in the sand trap.

To stay hydrated, drink about 4 ounces of plain water or sports drink every 15 to 20 minutes. If you're worried about nature calling while you're out there on the course, stick with a sports drink. The small amount of salt in the drink will encourage your body to retain fluid, decreasing the frequency of your need to urinate.

Strength for Your Swing

Although golf is not as rigorous as some other sports such as running, you do burn calories while playing. Depending on your body size, walking speed, club-carrying efforts, and course length, expect to use up at least 200 calories per hour.

Your body has plenty of stored energy to handle these energy needs in the

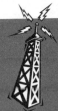

Nutrition News Flash

When you're out on the links for hours, you're bound to get a tad too much sun even if you wear sunscreen. Studies show that few people apply enough of the stuff, leaving themselves vulnerable to the sun's damaging rays. And not many people reapply the protection after a few hours like they should. Fortunately, you do have a second line of defense to protect you from skin cancer and premature aging: ketchup.

Ketchup and other processed tomato products contain high amounts of the antioxidant lycopene, one of the many plant pigments in the carotene family. When German researchers asked 20 volunteers to take a carotene supplement or a placebo, those who consumed the supplement were less likely to develop sunburn.

Carotene, a type of antioxidant found in brightly colored fruits and vegetables, may save your skin by binding to oxidized molecules, preventing them from damaging your skin. You can consume the amount of carotene that proved effective in the study by eating two processed tomato products each day.

Eating Smart for...
A Day on the Greens

Here's a typical day of meals to help you survive your next all-day golf tournament.

Early Morning
One breakfast bar
One banana
6 ounces orange juice
1 cup of coffee

The Front Nine
1 ounce trail mix (raisins, banana chips, sunflower seeds)
8 ounces sports drink

Lunch at the Clubhouse
One turkey club sandwich (two slices whole grain bread, 3 ounces roasted turkey, tomato and lettuce, 1 teaspoon reduced-fat mayonnaise, 1 teaspoon mustard)
½ cup bean salad
1 cup fruit salad (pears, apples, grapes)
Glass of iced tea

The Back Nine
One energy bar
16 ounces sports drink

Dinner
4 ounces grilled fish
1 cup risotto
1 cup green beans
2 cups greens
One slice of fruit tart

Calories: 1,840; Protein: 79 grams; Carbohydrate: 300 grams; Fat 21% calories

form of glycogen (carbohydrate) and fat. You may not have to worry about starving to death while on the course, but you do have to worry about low blood sugar levels. And after several hours, eating is crucial to maintain your circulating blood sugar levels.

You usually eat every few hours, even when you're sitting at your desk at work. On the course, you're walking for miles and standing for hours. As your muscles and brain pull sugar out of your bloodstream, your liver falls behind on replacing it. Once your blood sugar falls, you lose your ability to concentrate, and can even become shaky and light-headed.

To prevent a blood sugar drop, munch on fresh or dried fruit or a light sandwich, or drink 16 ounces of sports drink every 2 to 4 hours to stay energized.

Keeping Your Mind in the Game

When you play golf, you want to feel calm, cool, and collected. If you're not relaxed, you won't be able to concentrate and your swing will suffer. One sure way to lose your calm and focus is to consume too much caffeine or alcohol.

Caffeine

Caffeine from coffee, tea, or soda can cause feelings of anxiety. That, along with even the slightest trembling or shaking, can take the control out of your swing. If you're not a veteran coffee drinker, you're better off leaving the java alone. But if you drink a lot of coffee, you don't want to kick the habit cold turkey on the day of a big game. In fact, avoiding caffeine on the day you play may cause a performance disaster.

Caffeine acts as a stimulant, making you feel more awake. The catch is that your body easily becomes addicted. A caffeine jolt in the morning, for example, is a necessity for many people. But if you go without your regular dose, withdrawal symptoms like headache and lethargy kick in within a few hours. And the last thing you want on the golf course is an aching head and low energy.

If drinking coffee or some other caffeinated beverage is part of your daily routine, either set your mind to abstain completely or make the effort to reduce your everyday intake. And certainly don't increase your caffeine intake on the day of a game. If you plan to quit, don't do it cold turkey. Instead, cut your regular dose with half decaf. When your body has adapted to the reduced amount of caffeine, switch to tea, which has even less caffeine. Finally, switch to an herbal tea, which has no caffeine at all.

Alcohol

I don't know how beer and golf ever became linked in players' minds. The game takes the same amount of concentration as chess, and you don't see Bobby Fisher sitting at the chessboard with a frosty mug beside him.

If you want to keep your focus, there couldn't be a worse thing to drink than alcohol. It slows your reaction time and impairs your judgment—and you need plenty of both when you're out on the course. If you just can't separate your golf game from your beer, then you're better off celebrating your victory with a drink afterward, instead of imbibing while on the course.

If you still can't leave the clubhouse without a cold one close at hand, at least alternate your gulps of beer with draws from a bottle of sports drink to avoid dehydration.

Concentrate
on Yoga

My friends who practice yoga tell me that when they're trying to find inner calm they sometimes get distracted by their stomachs.

There are two problems that are most commonly associated with practicing yoga. The first and definitely most embarrassing is gas. Certain yoga positions put extra pressure on your abdomen at the same time that you are relaxing. Sometimes you're in an inverted position. Combine these moves with the high-fiber or vegetarian diets of many yoga practitioners, and you have the perfect recipe for gas.

Beyond gas, many of my friends who practice yoga tell me that they are trying to achieve a feeling of oneness through meditation. Eating the wrong foods can give them that not-quite-right feeling, however, which destroys their concentration.

Gas: No Laughing Matter

Everybody passes gas, both as burping and as flatulence. Each of us produces daily about ¾ liter of different gases in our intestinal tracts, mostly carbon dioxide, oxygen, hydrogen, and methane. Most gas is passed as flatulence, typically as many as 14 times a day. Excessive gas production can be both uncomfortable and embarrassing, especially in the middle of a quiet meditation during a yoga class.

workout q&a

Q: How can I make my gas less offensive?

A: Everyone's gas smells; to what degree depends on what you eat. You have millions of bacteria in your colon. These bacteria break down indigestible carbohydrate called oligosaccharides, which are typically found in beans, broccoli, and other high-fiber foods. As these fiber eaters do their work, they produce carbon dioxide, hydrogen, and methane gases, which you eventually pass out of your colon.

If you find excessive flatulence and its odor embarrassing, watch what you eat. If your diet is high in fiber or in oligosaccharide-rich foods such as lentils and other beans, you will produce more gas and the odor may be more pungent. Your best bet is to pinpoint the offending foods and eat less of them when you want to keep your flatulence under control. You can do that by keeping a diary of what you eat and when you pass gas.

Belches are primarily a result of gases that are released when you swallow air (this swallowing is called aerophagia) and to a lesser extent from gases in carbonated beverages. You swallow air by eating rapidly, chewing with your mouth open, or drinking beverages through straws. Aerophagia also occurs inadvertently when you swallow your saliva. For a few individuals, aerophagia is a nervous habit that may develop as a means to assuage feelings of hunger or to avert boredom. To stop ingesting air this way, examine how you chew and how fast you eat.

Flatulence, on the other hand, results from fermentation—the chemical breakdown of substances in food by the bacteria that live in your lower intestine or colon. The carbohydrate found in beans, broccoli, onions, and other vegetables and fruits makes wonderful fodder for colon bacteria. The end result is a whole lot of hydrogen, carbon dioxide, and methane gas.

There are many different kinds of bacteria, and the amount and type of gas produced depends on the mix of bacteria in your colon. Factors that influence colon bacteria populations have an impact on your gas production. Using antibiotics, eating yogurt or other foods with live bacterial cultures, and consuming high amounts of fiber all can alter the bacteria profile in your intestines. Here are some solutions to curb excess gas production.

Limit your lactose intake. Many people are unable to completely digest the milk sugar, or lactose, found in dairy products. The colon bacteria happily ferment the lactose, forming gas and giving you a bloated feeling. The over-the-counter products that aid in milk digestion work for many lactose-intolerant people.

Avoid large amounts of sorbitol and mannitol. Called sugar alcohols, sorbitol and mannitol are used to sweeten sugarless gums, candies, and other sugar-free products. These sugar alcohols are slowly digested, so when large amounts are consumed, such as eating a pint or more of sugar-free ice cream, sorbitol and mannitol are fermented by colon bacteria, causing gas and abdominal distension and discomfort.

Eat small meals. If you eat a high-fiber diet or are particularly partial to beans, broccoli, and cabbage (foods that are notorious for producing gas), you are better off eating small meals rather than gorging on larger amounts. By consuming smaller amounts of these gas-forming foods throughout the day, you'll produce less gas. Your production of gas rises after a large meal, as does your discomfort.

Vary your favorite high-fiber foods. Try different types of beans, vegetables, and fruits; some may be less gas-forming than others. By altering your diet, you'll not only lessen gas production but also increase the number of different nutrients you're taking in.

Try Beano. Available over-the-counter, Beano contains an enzyme that breaks down certain kinds of carbohydrate in foods such as beans and cabbage that our intestines barely touch but bacteria go wild over. A few drops on your first spoonful of lentil soup or forkful of broccoli should limit gas production in your colon.

Food and Focus

Don't let your meal interfere with your meditation. During yoga, you want a clear, relaxed mind. That's hard to achieve if your stomach is growling or if you just don't feel quite right.

Eating Smart for...
A Gas-Free Yoga Class

Try this day's worth of low-gas foods to avoid troublesome rumblings during your yoga session.

Breakfast
One slice whole wheat bread spread with 1 tablespoon apple butter
1 cup Cheerios topped with 2 tablespoons chopped apricots
6 ounces 1% milk
8 ounces orange juice

Lunch
Veggie burger on a whole wheat bun with tomato slices, lettuce, and sliced mozzarella cheese
10 baby carrots
1 ounce corn chips
Four gingersnap cookies

Afternoon Snack
1 ounce almonds
8 ounces cranberry juice

Dinner
1 cup penne pasta tossed with 3 ounces cooked shrimp and 2 tablespoons grated Parmesan cheese
¾ cup polenta
½ cup steamed asparagus
2 cups dark greens with ½ grated carrot and 1 tablespoon olive oil dressing
¾ cup chocolate sorbet

Calories: 2,480; Protein: 95 grams; Carbohydrate: 377 grams; Fat: 26% calories

Eating for yoga requires a careful balance of the right foods at the right time. Eat immediately before class, and you'll feel heavy and downright nauseated during some of the moves, especially inverted postures such as Shoulder Stands and the Downward Dog. If you eat too little food before class, your stomach may rumble, distracting you from your meditation. Here are a few pointers.

- If you practice a gentle form of yoga first thing in the morning, you may be able to get away with eating nothing. If you feel too weak on an empty stomach, drink a glass of juice or sports drink before you begin.
- If you practice yoga in the evening, eat a small snack during the middle of the afternoon. This will give you plenty of time to digest it so that it doesn't come back up during a Shoulder Stand, but not so much time that you'll feel hungry during class. Try a handful of pretzels, a few cubes of cheese, or a slice of bread spread with some hummus.
- Keep your diet relatively consistent. If you don't eat much meat, don't have a steak before class. Watch out for high-salt meals that may dehydrate you and leave you feeling less than your best.
- Avoid caffeine and alcohol just before your class. While they're perfectly legal, both of these substances are strong drugs that can affect your concentration and calm.

Run a Race

Whether you're running a 10-K or speedwalking for charity, you need to eat smart the whole week and the night before your big effort. Smart eating will fuel your muscles for the challenge as well as stockpile nutrients in your body for a faster recovery.

The problem is that many competitors' nutritional habits fall apart the weeks and days before a big race. A result of both prerace nerves and travel, this poor eating can drastically affect your performance. To prevent such a letdown, I've pulled together a step-by-step road map for you to follow the week before your big event. First, here are some basic facts about a popular concept in running nutrition.

Carbo-Loading

You've heard about carbo-loading—the practice of eating lots of high-carbohydrate calories during the week before a big race. People used to carbo-load only for endurance races such as marathons. It has long been known that when physical activity lasts more than 90 minutes, carbo-loading helps to maintain glycogen stores in the muscles. But research shows that carbo-loading works for shorter races as well.

In a study done by exercise physiologists from Texas Christian University in Fort Worth and the University of Toledo in Ohio, a group of trained runners were put on a high-carbohydrate diet (70 percent of calories) for 3 days before taking a treadmill test. The runners tapered their training for several days and rested the day before the test, just as they would before a race.

Compared to a standard diet of 40 percent carbohydrate, carboloading boosted performance in a high-intensity run lasting about 20 minutes. The athletes ran for 15 minutes at 75 percent of their maximum effort, then ran at their maximum effort for as long as possible. Carboloading increased their endurance by about 8 percent.

If you usually run a 25-minute 5-K, this may mean that you could maintain your fastest kick for 2 minutes longer than you normally would. Increase your carbohydrate intake to 500 to 600 grams a day (2,000 to 2,400 calories' worth) and cut back on your training a few days before any race or longer effort.

You can estimate your carbohydrate needs by allotting 17 to 26 calories per pound of body weight, depending on your training intensity. This amounts to 2,500 to 4,000 calories for a 150-pound person. Your carbohydrate intake should total at least 60 percent of your total calories, or 450 grams or more a day for a 150-pound person who trains moderately. Keep your fat intake at 20 to 25 percent of your calories (60 to 90 grams) and protein at about 15 to 20 percent (90 to 150 grams) per day.

7 Days and Counting

And now for your step-by-step nutritional eating plan. If you're competing in a shorter race that will last an hour or less, start this plan at "4 Days to Go." If you're planning a marathon, century bike ride, or any other multihour event, start at "7 Days to Go."

7 Days to Go

Since you'll be tapering your training at this point, do the same with your diet. To avoid gaining weight, you need to bring your calorie intake down about 100 calories for every mile you deduct from your training during your taper. You still want your carbohydrate intake to be sufficient to keep your glycogen stores full for race day, however.

workout q&a

Q: I have a tough time re-creating what I eat at home for a race that's away from home. I almost always end up at a restaurant, where I stuff myself. Even when I order pasta, I also have buttery garlic bread or some other high-fat fare. How can I keep myself in line?

A: When you get into town, look for a restaurant that serves familiar foods. No matter how much the travel guide has trumpeted the local sushi or Burmese joint, you're looking for old standbys. You can try riskier foods after the race. Find a restaurant that serves staples such as bread, baked potatoes topped with steamed veggies, and pasta with a light sauce.

After dinner, find a grocery or convenience store where you can stock up on breakfast items. My favorite is a banana or orange, a plain bagel, and a meal-replacement or -supplement drink such as SlimFast or Boost. This type of drink is easy on your stomach and travels well in an overnight bag. Other good choices are energy bars, carbohydrate gels, and packaged applesauce.

If you choose to eat out on race morning, stick with staples such as breakfast cereal, toast, oatmeal, or pancakes. Leave the hefty omelette or eggs Benedict for your postrace celebration.

Go for low-fat, high-carbohydrate foods such as whole grain cereal, bread, and pasta along with plenty of vegetables and fruit. Consider taking a multivitamin/mineral supplement that supplies 100 percent of the Daily Value (DV) to ensure an adequate intake, particularly if you tend to eat processed or packaged foods that may fall short on good nutrition. Over the next few days, be sure not to stuff yourself, but eat enough so that you don't feel hungry. It's especially important now to not skip meals.

4 Days to Go

For shorter races, begin your nutritional taper at this point. Cut back slightly on your calorie intake as you decrease your mileage these few days before the race. Since shorter races (less than an hour) don't tax your glycogen stores nearly as much as longer efforts do, carbohydrate intake is not as crucial. You'll want to keep carbohydrate intake at about 60 percent of your total calories, or roughly 450 grams of carbohydrate per day.

If you're a long distance athlete, you'll want to begin increasing your carbohydrate intake to 65 percent or more of total calories. This translates to almost 500 grams per day. If you don't have the appetite for that much pasta and potatoes, try liquid sources of carbohydrate such as fruit juices or sports drinks. And as you boost your carbohydrate intake, cut back slightly on fat and protein. Keep in mind that eating 500 grams of carbohydrate a day requires you to be a fat sleuth because too much fat will crowd out needed carbohydrate.

3 Days to Go

You've pared down your training, and you may be starting to feel a little sluggish. That's because your body responds to the training taper and the flood of carbohydrate by packing your muscles with more glycogen than usual. Since water gets tucked away along with the glycogen in your muscles, you may gain a little weight.

2 Days to Go

Many people break down nutritionally during the 2 days before a race. Often, this happens because you need to travel to a race, which changes your routine and makes it hard to stay on a steady eating schedule. And when you do eat, you have less control over how your food is prepared than you would at home. It's tougher to stay on top of fluid needs as well.

Minimize these pitfalls by planning ahead. If you're traveling, find out about restaurants and grocery stores near your hotel. Take along non-perishable, high-carbohydrate items such as energy bars, granola bars, sports drinks, cereal, and dried fruit, which are all great for augmenting your diet. For longer races, continue to keep carbohydrate intake at 500 to 600 grams a day; for shorter races, around 450 grams should do it.

Since heavy sweat loss during longer races leads to dehydration, you'll want to load up on fluids starting 2 days before your race. Drink plenty of liquids and make sure that your urine color is pale yellow or clear, not dark amber. (This is a simple but effective measure of adequate hydration.) Consuming sports drinks is a good way to get both fluids and carbohydrate.

This close to your race, you'll want to stay away from certain items. Beware of alcohol, especially if you'll be in a longer race. Alcohol interferes with glycogen and carbohydrate metabolism in your liver, which will shortchange your endurance. It also acts as a diuretic, or dehydration accelerator. Limiting high-fiber foods such as bran cereal, beans, and gas-producing vegetables will help keep bowel problems at bay. Stick with foods that agree with you.

The Day before a Race

You may think that if you eat only a little bit or not at all the day before a race, you will feel light on your feet, but skimping on food the day before only saps your precious glycogen stores. In less than 24 hours of fasting, you can completely drain your liver's supply of glycogen without any exercise. Skipping dinner the night before can hamper your race performance because your body burns carbohydrate even while you're asleep.

Be sure to rest, eat without stuffing yourself, and drink plenty of fluids. If you've been eating enough and sticking to high-carbohydrate fare that is modest in fat and protein, your glycogen stores will be at their peak by the end of this day. Snack frequently and stay with familiar foods. And just to be safe—especially if you're on the road—carry your own water bottle and drink from it often to stay hydrated.

Give careful consideration to the meal you eat on the night before your race. It should have 800 to 1,000 calories and should be high in carbohydrate and low in fat and protein. Avoid beans, broccoli, and other gas-causing foods, especially if they normally give you problems. Keep your meal low in fiber; you don't want to have to make frequent pit stops during the race. Keep alcohol to a strict minimum or skip it altogether. Finally, stick with your customary foods; the night before a race is not the time to experiment. The results could hinder your performance the next day.

On Race Day

A good rule of thumb is to eat a light meal the morning of your race. Consuming carbohydrate, particularly before longer races, provides en-

Recipe Revver

Night-before-the-Big-Race Hot Potato
Makes 1

More and more hotel rooms come equipped with microwave ovens, which makes smart eating the night before your race that much more convenient. Try the following in-room recipe, which contains easily packable items and goes great with a cornbread muffin and honey. Just stock up a cooler before you get to your hotel and be sure to bring along a set of utensils.

> 1 large potato
> 1½–2 cups fresh or frozen and thawed broccoli
> 2 ounces reduced-fat Cheddar cheese
> 8 ounces plain yogurt
> Salt and pepper

Pierce the potato in several places with a fork. Microwave the potato for 6 to 8 minutes or until tender. Microwave the broccoli for 1 to 2 minutes, or until just soft. Slice the potato in half and top with the cheese and ½ cup of the yogurt. Blend with a fork. Top with the broccoli and add one more dollop of yogurt. Season to taste with the salt and pepper.

Per potato: 634 calories, 16 g total fat, 10 g saturated fat, 40 g protein, 85 g carbohydrate, 14 g dietary fiber, 54 mg cholesterol, 730 mg sodium

ergy for hard-working muscles. Eat your prerace meal 2 to 4 hours before starting time. It should consist of at least 200 grams of carbohydrate, which works out to about 800 calories. For short events, you need only 300 to 600 calories.

To speed digestion, select foods and beverages that are low in fat and fiber. If you're worried about swings in your blood sugar levels, research shows that this has no ill effects on performance. Bagels, raisins, bananas, sports drink, pasta, and rice are great prerace foods. But if the thought of eating in those prerace morning hours doesn't sit well with your stomach, consider downing a liquid meal of sports drink, high-carbohydrate beverage, or nutritional supplement drink.

twenty-two

Finish a Marathon

Congratulations for taking on the marathon, possibly the greatest symbol of determination and chutzpah in a runner's career. Many people treat the marathon with reverence, as if all marathon finishers were superhuman. But finishing a marathon is not as difficult as you might think, as long as you train for it.

I like to think of the marathon as a metaphor for every challenging task in life. The way to conquer the marathon (and all of those other challenges) is to break it into small pieces and accomplish each piece one at a time. With the right training plan and determination, you can finish a marathon. That last 10-K might hurt a bit, but if the marathon were too easy, you would have nothing to brag about to your friends afterward.

Here's how to combine a nutrition and training program to fuel every step of your challenge.

Your Running Program

The key to completing your first marathon lies not in running scores of miles every week, but in one important weekly long run. Most runners do this long run on a weekend because that's when they have time to do it. Here are some rules to run by.

1. Pick a goal marathon roughly 6 months from now and sign up for it. If you don't have your entry in hand, you'll be much more likely to change your mind when the going gets tough.

2. Start this weekend with a long run that's 1 mile longer than your longest current run. For example, if you are currently running a maximum of 6 miles, start with a 7-mile long run. Write that run distance on your calendar. For the next 3 weekends, add a mile at a time to that long run. On the 4th weekend, cut that mileage in half for a recovery week. The following week, add another mile, and so on, until you reach 20 to 22 miles. Your first 2 months might look like this.

Week One: 7 miles	Week Five: 10 miles
Week Two: 8 miles	Week Six: 11 miles
Week Three: 9 miles	Week Seven: 12 miles
Week Four: 4.5 miles	Week Eight: 6 miles

3. Plan for a taper. You should complete your final 20-mile run at least 3 weeks before your marathon. That allows the small nicks and sore spots in your muscles time to mend before the big race. It also encourages your muscles to stockpile carbohydrate and small amounts of fat to burn during the marathon. To taper, cut your long run and weekly mileage in half each of the 3 weeks leading up to the race.

   For example, if you ran a total of 40 miles with a weekly long run of 20 miles 3 weeks before the marathon, your taper would look like this.

   2 weeks before
   Long run of 10 miles
   Total of 20 miles for the week

   1 week before
   No run longer than 5 miles
   Total weekly mileage of 10 miles

workout q&a

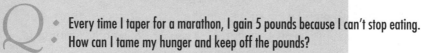

Q: Every time I taper for a marathon, I gain 5 pounds because I can't stop eating. How can I tame my hunger and keep off the pounds?

A: It's normal to expect some weight gain with a taper. With rest, your muscles get the signal to store up extra glycogen, which is part of the reason you taper. But since water gets packed away in your muscles along with the glycogen, you'll put on a few pounds as a result. Not much of that weight is from bulging fat cells.

Nevertheless, eat smart. As you decrease your mileage, you need to take in fewer calories, too—about 100 calories for every mile you cut. That sounds easy enough, but you may experience a ravenous appetite during your taper because your body treats this period as an opportunity to restock fuel stores of both glycogen and fat cells.

Stop your hunger pangs by filling up on foods that don't add tons of unwanted calories. Studies show that eating soups, fruits, and vegetables help people feel fuller, compared to lightweight snack foods such as chips and crackers that are loaded with calories.

4. Plan for at least one run of 20 miles. If you simply want to finish the marathon comfortably—which is a fine goal for your first marathon—then do only one 20-mile run. If you'd like to finish with a specific time, do two or more. If you're worried about running less than the total 26.2-mile distance, remember that you'll have fresh legs on marathon day.

Training Your Belly

As soon as you begin your marathon training, you need to start training your stomach and gastrointestinal (GI) tract to handle food on the run, especially if you've never consumed calories during exercise before.

As you run, your body drains stored carbohydrate from your muscles. After about 90 minutes, your body runs out of this fuel. As your muscles pull sugar out of your bloodstream, your liver attempts to replace it, but soon runs out of glycogen itself. Once your blood sugar falls, you'll feel weak, light-headed, and nauseated.

To prevent these problems, eat 100 calories of an easily digestible high-carbohydrate food (such as a banana or 12 ounces of sports drink) every half-hour to keep your blood sugar levels high. This isn't always easy. As you run, blood is diverted from your intestinal tract to your working muscles. This diversion decreases the efficiency of your stomach and intestines, making them less able to absorb fuel and fluid. As a result, fluids and food remain unprocessed, causing cramping and nausea.

Some people are more susceptible to GI upset than others. If you have a hard time digesting food at first, don't give up; over time, your stomach and GI tract will probably adapt. Start with sports drink and take small, frequent sips to prevent putting a huge load of fluid into your stomach at once. Look for those that contain mostly glucose and sucrose instead of fructose, which is absorbed more slowly than other sugars and may cause sloshing in your stomach.

Sports drinks do have some drawbacks. The bottles are usually too unwieldy to carry with you during training runs, and when you do run your marathon, you're at the mercy of the sports drink that the race officials decide to serve on the course. That's why some runners opt for energy gels and bars, which are easier to carry. Whatever form of nourishment you decide to consume, follow these tips for easy digestion and transport.

Stick with carbohydrate. Fat and protein slow digestion, so eat high-carbohydrate foods.

Learn the right mix. If you choose energy bars or gels, you need to drink water with them to wash the calories through your stomach and into your intestines. Make sure you drink 4 to 8 ounces of water with each bar or gel pack.

Train with the sports drink you'll have on race day. For promotional purposes, many sports drink companies donate their drinks to races. But you have no way to know what drink will be served until long after you've registered for your race. You want to minimize the number of variables on race day, so keep tabs on race officials until they announce what drink is going to be served during the race, then train with it.

Be creative. It's tough to carry enough sports drink with you to last an entire 20-mile run. Instead, you can run 5-mile loops around a car fully stocked with sports drink and stop at every pass to refuel, have a friend accompany you on a bike that's loaded with sports drink, or stash bottles along your course beforehand.

Your Training Diet

Many people think that once they start training for a marathon, they can eat whatever they want because they are burning so many calories. They couldn't be more misguided.

First, not everyone burns more calories when they train for a marathon. That 20-mile run may add up to 2,000 incinerated calories, but if you don't increase your overall weekly mileage, you won't burn more calories than when you weren't marathon training. In fact, you may scale back your other runs during the week when you start adding miles on the weekend because your long run will make your muscles ache. You'll want more rest days than before.

In other words, if you ran 30 miles a week before you began training for the marathon, and you continue to run 30 miles a week during marathon training, pigging out will only make you gain weight.

Second, marathon training taxes your muscles, joints, tendons, energy levels, and immunity. Numerous studies show that free radical formation increases after an exhausting run. And in one study, runners who finished a half-marathon had more free radical damage than they did before the run. Fortunately, you can do something to prevent this.

Your body has a natural defense system that partially protects you against free radical damage. Each cell contains a variety of antioxidant enzymes with names like SuperOxide Dismutase (SOD). These enzymes extinguish many of the "fires" caused by free radicals. As you become more fit, your body increases the activity of these antioxidant enzymes. But these enzymes do only part of the job. Antioxidants from the foods you eat provide the rest of your natural defense. Here's how to use these nutrients to your advantage.

Bump up your vegetable intake. Nutrients such as carotenoids (substances that your body converts to vitamin A) and vitamins C and E are found abundantly in fruits and vegetables. These nutrients neutralize free radicals. Green, leafy vegetables; citrus fruits; carrots; and other kinds of fruits and vegetables are packed with these protective substances. Eat eight or more servings each day of as many different fruits and vegetables as you can.

Eight servings may sound like a lot, but a cup of leafy greens, ½ cup of chopped vegetables, 6 ounces of vegetable or fruit juice, or any piece of fruit counts as a serving. Include produce at every meal by putting fruit on cereal, layering sliced vegetables on sandwiches, making salads, and adding vegetables to every dish you cook.

Get plenty of minerals. You can strengthen your body's natural antioxidant enzymes with minerals such as zinc, manganese, and copper. You'll find these in whole grains, meats, seafood, and fortified breakfast cereals.

Focus on vitamins C and E. Taking supplements may provide an additional antioxidant edge that you can't get from eating a healthful diet. There are many antioxidant supplements on the market, but studies show that vitamins C and E may be the most effective. By supplementing with these vitamins, you're creating auxiliary antioxidant defenses throughout your body.

In addition to preventing disease down the road, supplements may prevent short-term problems like muscle soreness. Taking 400 IU of vitamin E and 250 to less than 1,000 milligrams of vitamin C is safe and may prove beneficial.

Eat enough carbohydrate. Some research suggests that getting enough of this important macronutrient during heavy training may also boost your immunity. Try to consume 60 percent of your calories from carbohydrate, 25 percent from fat, and 15 percent from protein. For the average 2,800-calorie-per-day diet, that comes to 420 grams of carbohydrate, 77 grams of fat, and 105 grams of protein.

Go fish. Fish contains important fats that fight inflammation and boost immunity. Aim for two servings of a fatty cold-water fish such as salmon or mackerel each week.

Timing

When it comes to marathon performance, you should divide carbohydrate foods into two categories: quickly digested (high-glycemic) carbohydrate such as candy, and nutrient-packed, low-glycemic carbohydrate such as whole grains and produce, which is digested more slowly. Knowing when to eat which type can make a huge impact on the success of your training. Eat too much high-glycemic carbohydrate, and you won't get enough nutrients to keep your muscles healthy. Eat too many low-glycemic carbohydrate foods, and you may not recover as quickly as you would like. To make sure that you eat the right foods at the right times and in the right amounts, follow these tips.

Plan carbohydrate feasts around your long runs. High-glycemic foods should be the mainstay of your meals before and after your long runs. Any type of sugary, nonfat food (apple juice, jelly beans, licorice), some refined grains (pasta, white rice, white bread), and even whole wheat bread, potatoes, and corn count as high-glycemic foods.

Aim for 200 to 300 grams of carbohydrate (800 to 1,200 calories) 3 to 4 hours before your long run. (If you run first thing in the morning, eat high-glycemic foods at your evening meal and then have a sports drink before heading out for your run.) For example, eat a pancake breakfast with plenty of syrup, a glass of orange juice, and an energy bar. Besides giving you quick energy, refined carbohydrate is almost always low in fiber, which prevents annoying pit stops during your run.

If you need a quick meal a half-hour before your run, aim for 30 to 60 grams of carbohydrate, or 120 to 240 calories. During your run, consume 30 to 60 grams of carbohydrate an hour.

After your long run, guzzle a sports drink or glass of fruit juice before you head for the shower. As soon as you're cleaned up, sit down to a meal that contains mostly high-glycemic foods with some protein, such as apple juice and a baked potato topped with cottage cheese.

Eat plenty of fruits, vegetables, and whole grains on your easy days. Since getting enough carbohydrate to fuel your muscles isn't as critical on these low-mileage or rest days, concentrate on packing in all the nutrition you missed when focusing on those high-glycemic, vitamin-vacant foods. On these days, eat whole grains such as quinoa, barley, millet, brown rice, slow-cooking oatmeal, whole wheat pastas, and cooked beans. Don't forget to pile on the fruits and vegetables.

The Last Supper

Go to a prerace clinic before any marathon, and I guarantee that you will hear someone ask, "What should I eat before the race?" It's the most-asked running question of them all.

At least it won't be you asking. If you follow my plan, your fluid and energy stores (primarily glycogen) will be fully stocked, and your vitamin and mineral levels will be at their peak on the morning of the race. Nutritionally, you'll be ready to run.

The Week before a Marathon

During the 7 days before your marathon, consume 2,500 to 4,000 total calories a day, or 17 to 26 calories per pound of body weight. You'll want to decrease your normal caloric intake somewhat since you won't be running as much. A good general rule is to subtract 100 calories for every mile you cut while tapering.

As for nutrient mix, consume 60 to 70 percent of your calories as carbohydrate, or 375 to 450 grams daily. This will ensure that your glycogen stores will be at their maximum. Keep fat at 20 to 30 percent of total calories (60 to 90 grams) and protein at 10 to 20 percent (80 to 110 grams).

- Eat a variety of high-carbohydrate foods. Along with bagels and pasta, get plenty of grains, fruits, and anything else that is high in energizing carbohydrate.
- Keep your meal and snack times regular; your digestive tract will thank you.
- Consider using carbohydrate-supplement products such as Gatorade Torq. They make it easier to get the nutrients you need, especially when you're traveling.

- Keep a close eye on food labels and stay away from high-fat foods.
- Don't skip meals. Skipping meals can drain your glycogen stores in a hurry.
- Don't stuff yourself. You want to feel light on your feet on race morning.
- Don't eat too much of any one food because it can play havoc with your intestines.

The Day before a Marathon

What you eat—and what you don't eat—the day before a marathon can have a big effect on your race performance. Your goals for this crucial day are to top off your glycogen tank, get well-hydrated, and avoid the kind of gut trouble that comes from eating the wrong foods.

Since you'll be resting and not burning many calories on this day, be careful that you don't eat too much; you'll feel sluggish if you do. Consume 2,000 to 3,500 calories, 65 to 70 percent of which should be carbohydrate. Eat small amounts throughout the day, which may mean taking portable food—energy bars, sandwiches, fruit, pretzels, or other wholesome snacks—with you when you leave your house or hotel room.

- Keep a water bottle with you at all times and drink from it frequently. Pale yellow or clear urine is a sign that you're well hydrated; darker yellow means that you need to drink more.
- Be conservative. Eat home-cooked meals (if possible) to avoid food poisoning.
- Don't eat gas-forming foods such as broccoli and beans on the night before the race.
- Don't overindulge in caffeinated beverages. They increase your urine output, which could leave you dehydrated.
- Don't overindulge in alcohol. Better yet, skip it altogether. It's a diuretic, and it can also hamper glycogen metabolism in your liver.

The Day of a Marathon

Before, during, and after a marathon, the right balance of carbohydrate and fluid is vital to your performance and recovery.

Eat a meal 2 to 4 hours before race time. If you don't, you'll experience early fatigue. Your race-day morning meal should consist of high-carbohydrate foods; aim for 100 to 200 grams of carbohydrate.

Drink about 16 ounces of fluid 2 hours before the start of the marathon. This will give you enough time to void any excess. Once the race starts, drink fluids and consume carbohydrate—liquid or solid—early and often. Your goal is to take in 5 to 12 ounces of fluid every 15 to 20 minutes, and 30 to 60 grams of carbohydrate (120 to 240 calories) every hour of running.

After a Marathon

Now that you've finished your marathon, forget what I said earlier about it not being that difficult. Right now, you should gloat; few people even attempt this distance.

You trained, you ran, and you finished. Congratulations.

Your body probably feels like it has been trampled by the other runners. To get back on your feet as soon as possible, go into nutrition-recovery mode immediately following the race. First, drink as much fluid as you can. Each pound you lose during a marathon—and most people lose several—includes 16 ounces of fluid loss.

To begin rebuilding your glycogen stores, eat 50 to 100 grams of carbohydrate within 30 minutes of finishing. Follow this up with about 50 grams of carbohydrate every 2 hours. You want to eventually consume about 600 grams of carbohydrate within the next 24 hours. This should fully restore your glycogen levels.

Eat a little protein right after finishing, too. Research has shown that protein may speed glycogen rebuilding. The sooner you restock your glycogen stores, the sooner you'll be back on the roads training for your next marathon.

Hold off on the fatty foods and alcohol. Gobbling burgers, greasy pizza, or fat-laden desserts will crowd out the carbohydrate you should be getting, which will slow your recovery and leave you feeling sluggish. (If you don't care about feeling sluggish, go right ahead and have that ice cream.) Complete refueling of your glycogen tanks takes about 24 hours and requires at least 2,400 calories of carbohydrate.

Eating Smart for...a Marathon

The Week before the Race

Use this menu and the following ones as guides. For example, try vegetarian chili instead of lentil soup for lunch. I list rice for dinner, but feel free to substitute a similar amount of pasta or potatoes; top it with fish, tofu, or a type of meat other than turkey if you wish, but stick to the serving size.

Breakfast
2 cups Wheaties or other whole grain cereal
8 ounces 1% milk
1 cup sliced strawberries
Two slices whole wheat toast spread with 1 tablespoon honey

Lunch
1 cup lentil soup
Two cornbread muffins
1 cup carrot-raisin salad made with reduced-fat mayonnaise
Two large oatmeal cookies

Afternoon Snack
1 cup low-fat vanilla yogurt mixed with ¼ cup chopped dried apricots

Dinner
1½ cups rice topped with 4 ounces ground turkey
½ cup each of steamed broccoli and carrots
1 cup romaine salad with 2 tablespoons low-fat Italian dressing
Two 2-inch square marshmallow-rice treats

Calories: 3,000; Protein: 103 grams; Carbohydrate: 480 grams; Fat: 23% calories

The Day before the Race

It's almost here. Don't experience an 11th-hour nutritional letdown; keep eating smart.

Breakfast
Two 7-inch pancakes topped with 2 tablespoons syrup
4 ounces orange juice

Morning Snack
1 cup low-fat vanilla yogurt mixed with 1 sliced banana

Lunch
Turkey sandwich (two slices whole wheat bread, 2 ounces sliced turkey, 1 ounce cheese,
1 teaspoon mustard)
1 cup grapes
Small frozen yogurt cone

Afternoon Snack
One energy bar
16 ounces sports drink

Dinner
One large baked potato topped with ½ cup low-fat cottage cheese
½ cup steamed carrots
One sourdough roll

Evening Snack
1 cup cornflakes
4 ounces fat-free milk

Calories: 2,400; Protein: 92 grams; Carbohydrate: 450 grams; Fat: 12% calories

Race Day

Always eat on the morning of a race to bolster your carbohydrate stores.

Breakfast
One toasted plain bagel with 2 tablespoons jam
One banana
½ cup rice sprinkled with cinnamon
8 ounces sports drink

Calories: 550; Protein: 11 grams; Carbohydrate: 127 grams; Fat: 3% calories

(continued)

Eating Smart for...a Marathon (cont.)

During the Race

In addition to eating these fueling extras, make sure you drink plenty of water at all stations along the route.

Mile 6
   8 ounces sports drink

Mile 12
   1½ cubes guava paste (or substitute your own proven energy booster)

Mile 15
   8 ounces sports drink

Mile 17
   One energy gel pack

Mile 21
   8 ounces sports drink

Calories: 400; Protein: 0 grams; Carbohydrate: 100 grams; Fat: 0% calories

Immediately following the Race

The following foods will help speed your recovery if eaten within 30 minutes after finishing a marathon.

   One energy bar
   One soft pretzel
   16 ounces sports drink

Calories: 515; Protein: 10 grams; Carbohydrate: 105 grams; Fat: 5% calories

1½ Hours following the Race

This is the type of meal you should eat to help recover from running a marathon.

   2 cups Asian noodles tossed with 4 ounces grilled chicken
   ⅓ cup each snow peas, broccoli, and carrots
   1 cup rice pudding topped with ½ cup sliced strawberries
   12 ounces fruit juice

Calories: 1,278; Protein: 59 grams; Carbohydrate: 167 grams; Fat: 31% calories

chapter twenty-three

Ride a Century

So, you're taking on the century? Although it's not technically a race, this 100-mile effort usually marks an important stage in a cyclist's life, much like the marathon does for a runner, an Ironman does for a triathlete, and a mile or 2-mile effort does for a swimmer. Sure, there are longer races; there's cross-country riding, where people average 80 to 140 miles every day. The century, however, is still the most popular and revered goal.

Preparing for a century requires just as much nutritional know-how in the kitchen as it does physical training on the bike. Here's how to master both areas for a successful ride.

Readying Your Body

To train for a century, I recommend a 10-week program where you concentrate on one long ride a week. If this is your first century, start with a long ride of about 30 miles (unless you've already ridden longer distances) and add 4 to 5 miles a week until you reach 60 miles. This will allow you to finish comfortably in 8 to 10 hours.

If you're planning on riding a stronger, faster century, start with a 40-mile weekly long ride and work your way up to about 75 miles. The rest of your weekly rides should range from easy 6-mile spins to longer 20- to 30-mile rides. All totaled, your weekly mileage should grow from an early-

workout q&a

Q:
I would like to train for a century, but my busy schedule sometimes prevents me from training. What should I do?

A:
If you have trouble finding time for all of the rides you need for training, try the following.

Commute to work. This is the single best way to fit in mileage. Also, consider riding your bike just about everywhere you need to go, from visiting a friend to a quick trip to the store. You can carry a change of clothes in a backpack.

Ride on a stationary trainer. If you can't get out on the roads because you have small children to keep an eye on, get in your miles on a stationary trainer. If you want to take advantage of a beautiful day, set up the trainer in your driveway or yard and ride while the children play nearby.

Spin. Because they pack a lot of high intensity into a short amount of time, Spinning classes at the gym are a great way to get in shape for a century. Just don't substitute them for your longest ride of the week.

season 70 to 100 miles a week to an event-ready 180 total weekly miles.

Why not ride long every time you hop in the saddle? For one, most people don't have the time. Second, your body will benefit most from different types of training. The short, easy spins will help warm up your legs, easing muscle soreness and giving your legs needed practice in pedaling at a faster rate than usual. You can use other rides to build skills you'll need for the race. For example, if the race is hilly, make sure some of your training rides include tough climbing.

To help your legs (especially your knees) survive the long ride, keep the bike in a lower gear so that you can pedal at a rate of 85 to 90 revolutions per minute. Practice the subtle art of pedaling in perfect circles by pulling up on the pedal as much as you push down. Try removing one foot from its toeclip so that you're pedaling with only one foot. Wherever you feel an awkward slackness is where you need to practice pedaling with more of a circular motion.

During the week before the race, you'll want to taper for the big event. You may worry that all of your long months of training will slip away, but that's not the case. In fact, during these last few days, your body is busy repairing any nicks and dents in your muscles as well as stocking your fuel tanks for the big day. Of all the aspects of training, the taper is perhaps the most important.

Readying Your Belly

Eating smart for your upcoming 100-mile ride is just as important as training. As your rides get longer and your weekly mileage grows, you need more carbohydrate and protein in your diet. During long rides, your muscles burn stored glycogen. You must replace your reserves of carbohydrate energy before you hop back in the saddle; otherwise, you'll bonk quickly.

An inactive person needs about 300 grams of carbohydrate daily. Because you're training, you need 400 to 600 grams, depending on your mileage, so eat at least 1,600 calories of carbohydrate each day.

A great time to get a big dose of carbohydrate is right after a training ride, when your muscles are ready to rebuild spent glycogen stores. Aim to eat 100 to 150 grams of carbohydrate within an hour after each ride. Here are some good snacks in that range.

- One banana, one energy bar, and 8 ounces sports drink
- A tuna sandwich, 1 cup pasta salad, and 1 cup fruit salad
- 1½ cups pasta tossed with tomato sauce, one fig bar, and 8 ounces fat-free milk
- 2 ounces pretzels, two oatmeal cookies, one mozzarella cheese stick, and 8 ounces fruit juice
- 1½ cups cereal, 8 ounces fat-free milk, 2 tablespoons raisins, and one apple
- One bean burrito, 1 cup bean salad, and one orange

Throughout the day, focus on eating the following carbohydrate-rich foods that are also packed with key nutrients that your body needs for riding performance.

Fruits and vegetables. Eat 8 or more servings of fruits and vegetables every day. Try snacking on fresh or dried fruits, especially during longer bike rides when your muscles may be running low on stored glycogen.

Whole grains. Have 10 or more servings daily. Some easy ways to get grains into your diet include cereal in the morning and brown rice, pasta, or hearty whole grain bread for lunch, dinner, or even an evening snack.

Sports drinks and energy bars. In addition to a well-rounded diet, sports drinks and energy bars provide a convenient way to load up on carbohydrate. Check the labels for carbohydrate content.

Besides carbohydrate, your body will also need extra protein to rebuild muscle tissue. You need 90 to 125 grams daily, depending on your weight. To compute your needs more precisely, multiply your weight in pounds by 0.7 to get a recommended intake of protein in grams.

Some good sources (add at least one to every meal) are soy, seafood, lean meats, poultry, low-fat or fat-free dairy products, and bean-and-grain combinations like bean burritos. For reference, a 3-ounce serving of chicken has 21 grams of protein and a 3-ounce soy burger contains 15 grams.

You need to eat a lot of food to meet these carbohydrate and protein targets, but your calorie needs also increase during training. Try to eat at least six times daily—three or four meals and two or three snacks. Be sure to have one of those meals (or at least a hefty snack) soon after your ride, to replenish the fuel that your muscles need.

You'll also need more fluid (both during your training sessions and after) to offset sweat losses. For each half-hour you train, drink an additional 24 to 32 ounces of water during the day.

Staying Healthy

The longer you're on the road, the more air you breathe. That means more pollutants and more oxygen. You know what's wrong with breathing in carbon monoxide, but what could be wrong with oxygen? Plenty.

Even though your body needs oxygen to survive, this life-giving element can also be harmful, setting off a chain of events that can lead to inflammation, muscle soreness, and lowered immunity. Like cigarette smoke, smog, and other kinds of air pollution, oxygen can become destructive once inside your body. It turns into and promotes the growth of potentially harmful molecules called free radicals. These molecules are missing an electron, which makes them unstable. To stabilize themselves, free radicals pillage electrons from nearby proteins, genetic material, and protective cell structures.

Fortunately, antioxidants from the foods you eat can help stop their destructive search. In other words, during periods of heavy training, you need to eat more healthfully than ever. Unfortunately, many cyclists start eating poorly during these times because in one sense, they can get away with it. They are burning so many calories that foods that they once limited to control their weight are now fair game. That's fine, as long as you don't let beer, cheese, and pie crowd out the necessary staples of fruits and vegetables, minerals, and foods high in vitamins C and E.

Fueling for the Big Ride

Think of each training ride as a practice century. Find out what types of foods, fluids, amounts, and timing work best for you.

Experiment with taking breaks. You'll be taking breaks during the event, so you'll need to know the right intervals that work for you. Some riders take only one break for a midday meal. But if this is your first century, take a break at least once an hour. Experiment with what amount of food you can comfortably digest during that break and still be able to get back on your bike to ride. And use your breaks to stretch out your neck, shoulders, arms, and legs.

Learn to eat and drink in the saddle. It is imperative to learn how to reach for your water bottle without dropping it. To safely steer while grabbing for a water bottle, move one hand to the center of your handlebar. During your training, try no-handed drills to get used to balancing the bike with just your feet and legs. (If you are uncoordinated, stick with one-

My Food Diary

My training buddies often tease me about my affinity for tomato sandwiches. During every century, I pull into the rest area, grab two large slices of bread, smack some tomatoes between the slices, and start eating. People look at me askance until they find out that I'm a nutrition expert—and until I tell them how good the sandwich tastes. When you're tired, thirsty, and hungry, there's just something about a tomato sandwich that really hits the spot.

handed riding.) Because it's hard to open prepackaged foods while in the saddle, open them before the ride or tear a small portion of the packaging so that you can rip off the rest with your teeth.

Drink two bottles of water every hour. During the century, you can refill your water bottles at aid stations. On training rides, you'll need to find businesses or residences where you can refill. For sports drink, bring along premeasured powder in a resealable plastic bag to mix into your bottle.

Practice century-day nutrition ahead of time. You should never eat anything on the day of the century that you haven't tried during your training. If you plan to eat the food served at the aid stations, find out what foods will be served. If you don't plan to partake of the aid station food, make sure you can carry enough of your own in your jersey pockets.

The Week before a Century

During the 7 days before your century, allot yourself 2,500 to 4,000 calories a day, or 17 to 26 calories per pound of body weight. Consume 60 to 70 percent of your calories as carbohydrate to pack your glycogen stores to their maximum. Keep fat at 20 to 30 percent of calories (60 to 90 grams) and protein at 10 to 20 percent (65 to 100 grams). Follow these strategies to keep yourself in shape for the event.

- Eat a variety of high-carbohydrate foods; don't just focus on bagels or pasta for your carbohydrate needs.
- Keep your meal and snack times regular, and to avoid gastrointestinal (GI) upset, don't eat too much of any one food.
- If you're traveling to the event, pack some carbohydrate-supplement products such as Gatorade Torq. They make it easier to get the carbohydrate you need when you're surrounded by steakhouses.
- Keep a close eye on food labels, and stay away from high-fat foods.

The Day before a Century

What you eat—and don't eat—the day before a century can have a big effect on your performance. You want to top off your glycogen tank, get well-hydrated, and avoid a lot of fiber that could possibly make you take annoying pit stops during the event.

Since you won't be burning many calories the day before the century,

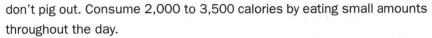

don't pig out. Consume 2,000 to 3,500 calories by eating small amounts throughout the day.

For your dinner the night before the event, aim for 800 to 1,000 calories, with the emphasis on carbohydrate. This meal should be low in fat, protein, and fiber, and it should include familiar foods that sit well in your stomach. Here are a few more tips to help keep you eating smart.

- Drink frequently during the day.
- Eat home-cooked meals (if possible) to avoid food poisoning.
- Limit your intake of caffeinated beverages. They'll increase your urine output and leave you dehydrated.
- Don't overindulge in alcohol; it's a diuretic, and it can also hamper glycogen metabolism in the liver.

The Day of the Century

The century is a long event, and you need sustenance to get through it. For starters, eat a meal 2 to 4 hours before start time. Skipping a meal will decrease your carbohydrate stores, and you'll experience fatigue early in the event. Your morning meal should consist of high-carbohydrate foods; aim for 100 to 200 grams of carbohydrate (400 to 800 calories). Drink about 16 ounces of fluid 2 hours before start time.

During the century, eat and drink liberally. You can handle only about 2 hours of steady riding without taking in some form of calories. After that, your muscles run out of stored carbohydrate and you slow down. Your goal is 5 to 12 ounces of fluid every 15 to 20 minutes, and 30 to 60 grams of carbohydrate (120 to 300 calories) during every hour.

Sports drinks offer a simple way to get the right amount of fluid and carbohydrate, and most of them come with the optimal proportion of both. Try to drain two bottles of sports drink an hour. Or try energy gels, energy bars, or bananas. Make sure you drink water, too.

Take advantage of the food served at the rest stops, but don't treat it as a chance to gorge. You should eat and drink during the race as you have during your training. Instead of waiting too long to take a break, take several very short breaks every hour. Don't break for longer than 10 minutes, however; if you do, you'll have a tough time getting started again.

Eating Smart for...a Century

Before the Race

From the moment you wake up on the day of the century, smart eating will give you an edge. Try this power-packed breakfast for a fast start.

Breakfast
> Three 6-inch pancakes
> 2 tablespoons jam or syrup
> One banana
> 6 ounces orange juice
> Cup of coffee

Calories: 650; Protein: 12 grams; Carbohydrate: 118 grams; Fat: 22% calories

During the Race

Feeding your body a steady supply of fuel is a must for the success of your attempt. Don't forget to stay hydrated by drinking water throughout the event.

Mile 20
> One banana
> 8 ounces sports drink

Mile 35
> One energy gel pack

Mile 52 (Lunch stop)
> Two slices bread with light filling (turkey, cheese slices, or jam)
> Two fig bars
> One apple
> 8 ounces sports drink

After the Ride

Recovery begins the moment you get off your bike. First, rehydrate yourself by drinking a generous amount of water. Next, rebuild your depleted glycogen stores by eating 50 to 100 grams of carbohydrate within 30 minutes of finishing. Follow this up with an average of 50 grams of car-

Mile 75
Three dried pear halves
16 ounces sports drink

Mile 90
Two fig bars
8 ounces sports drink

Calories: 1,130; Protein 18 grams; Carbohydrate: 260 grams; Fat: 7% calories

After the Race

Many organized rides offer a great recovery meal. Here's an example of what I ate after my century in the lava flats of Northern California near Mt. Shasta.

2 cups pasta with ¾ cup meat sauce
1 cup wild-rice salad
2 cups greens with chickpeas, cucumbers, 1 tablespoon oil and vinegar dressing
One slice of sourdough bread
12 ounces iced tea

Calories: 852; Protein: 25 grams; Carbohydrate: 160 grams; Fat: 18% calories

bohydrate every 2 hours; your goal is to consume about 2,400 calories—500 to 600 grams of carbohydrate—within the next 24 hours. Take in a little protein right after your ride, too, to speed your recovery and get you back on that bike training for your next century.

twenty-four

Hike
All Day

Because hiking usually involves spectacular views and soothing natural settings, many people are tricked into thinking that hikers need little more preparation than someone who's walking from their front door to their mailbox. This type of thinking can be extremely dangerous.

Flimsy footwear can lead to a violently twisted ankle. Cotton clothing offers no protection against a sudden downpour, or against overheating on a hot day. Unlike synthetic fabrics that wick sweat away from your skin and dry quickly, cotton tends to get soaked and stay soaked, which can easily make you too hot or too cold, depending on the elements. Not having a map means that there's a chance of getting lost. And when you get lost, lack of food and water can lead to low energy, dehydration, and even disaster.

So whether you plan to hike the steep inclines of beautiful Rocky Mountain National Park, the large boulders of the Appalachian Trail, or the wooded paths in your own backyard, you need to pay careful attention to the food and fluids you pack for your journey. Here's a look at what your body needs to carry you safely through an all-day hike.

Quenching Your Thirst

Fluids rank at the top of the list for any type of hike or walk that will last longer than a half-hour. As you trek over the trail, your body generates heat that must be dissipated so that your organs and muscles don't overheat and go into failure. Warm outside temperatures also prompt your body to sweat more in an effort to stay cool.

Under these conditions, you can easily lose about a liter of sweat per hour. Replenishing all of your sweat losses is ideal but hardly practical since you would have to haul 8 to 10 liters of water for a 5- to 8-hour hike—that's more than 18 pounds. Instead, pack one-half to two-thirds of this amount, or 4 to 6 liters. During your hike, drink about 250 milliliters (4 ounces) every 15 minutes. And when you finish your daylong effort, replenishing lost fluid is a priority.

You can carry water-filled bottles in a backpack or fanny pack. Or you may want to consider investing in a water backpack device, which works well for hiking and holds a substantial amount of water. Made by Camelbak, Nathan, and other companies, these backpacks have an inner bladder with a convenient tube and mouthpiece that enables hands-free drinking. Some styles have compartments for energy bars and trail mix.

Whatever you do, don't rely on natural sources of water to quench your thirst. While out in the woods, you may feel like you've left the evils of civilization behind, but you haven't. Because of pollution, there are few streams that are safe to drink from anymore. And you don't want to perform a personal experiment to find that out. The germs *giardia, cryptosporidium,* and others that lurk in running stream water can bring on a terrible case of diarrhea and cramping, which leads to dehydration—the problem you were trying to avoid in the first place.

If you plan to camp overnight and simply can't carry enough water, invest in a water filter or purifier. These gadgets are getting smaller and lighter; most cost $50 or less. You could also boil your water or treat it with iodine tablets, but the filter is the most convenient option.

Satisfying Your Hunger

Depending on the terrain, trail incline, weight of your pack, and hiking speed, you can easily burn 400 or more calories per hour. Your muscles burn stored carbohydrate energy, called glycogen, as well as stored fat. During several hours of hiking, your stores of glycogen can easily run out, leaving you feeling too drained to take another step, let alone get back to camp.

To avoid this problem, take along carbohydrate-rich foods and eat 150 to 200 calories every hour. Many of these foods are bulky, such as fruit and bread, making them impractical to carry. Try dried fruit such as raisins, apples, and papaya, which are loaded with the carbohydrate calories you need for the long haul.

You also need some satisfying food to provide fat and protein. And since fat packs more than twice as many calories per gram than carbohydrate does, taking along some nutritious, fat-rich food makes great sense. This is where trail mix comes in—a traditional hiker's food made of nuts, dried fruit, and other goodies such as soy nuts or—my favorite—chocolate chips. (They may melt at warmer temperatures, but they still taste good.)

Nuts also supply another hiking staple: salt. During a long hike, you can develop a rare but dangerous condition called hyponatremia. When you sweat out too much sodium or drink too much water (or, more likely, both), the sodium in your blood becomes diluted. This electrolyte imbalance causes a number of symptoms, from fatigue to dizziness to nausea to death. The symptoms are similar to dehydration, with one major difference: When you are dehydrated and you drink water, you tend to feel better quickly. When you have hyponatremia and you drink more water, you feel worse. Although drinking copious amounts of water can cause hyponatremia, don't opt for dehydration. Instead, consume some form of salt during your hike. The salt can come in the form of a sports drink or in your trail mix.

Research has found that ibuprofen inhibits your body's ability to dispose of excess fluid through urination. That can make it more likely that you'll come down with a case of hyponatremia, especially in hot weather. Skip the painkillers. Instead, ready your body for the trip with some healthy training in the great outdoors.

Here are some more nutritional tips for your hike.

Always pack more food than you need. You never know whether you'll be out on the trail longer than you expect. You could run into bad weather;

Recipe Revver
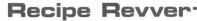

Healthy-Hiking Trail Mix
Makes 3⅓ cups

Most commercial trail mixes contain too much protein and fat for even moderate-intensity hiking. This recipe, however, gets a good dose of carbohydrate from the raisins and cranberries. Trail mix keeps for 6 to 8 weeks in the refrigerator.

1 cup whole almonds
1 cup dried cranberries
½ cup raisins
½ cup roasted soy nuts
¼ cup dry-roasted pumpkin seeds
¼ cup dried coconut (optional)

Combine the almonds, cranberries, raisins, nuts, seeds, and coconut (if using). Store the mix in a plastic container with a tight-fitting lid.

Per ⅓ cup: 180 calories, 8 g protein, 13 g carbohydrate, 11 g total fat, 2 g saturated fat, 0 mg cholesterol, 4 g dietary fiber, 0 mg sodium

take a long, scenic detour; or, in a worst-case scenario, injure yourself and have to wait for help to arrive. Always pack one extra meal just in case. And remember to pack out your trash. If everyone tossed their empty water bottles and energy bar wrappers where they walked, trails would no longer be beautiful places to hike. Pack out everything that you pack in. You can even bring an extra plastic bag to load up with the remains of previous litterbugs. The trail will thank you.

Learn to pack light. Your pack should weigh no more than 50 pounds. If you're on vacation, you may be carrying a little more than usual, such as a camera or binoculars. These items take up space in your pack and weigh quite a bit, so you'll have to make careful choices about what else you put into your bag. To make sure that you can carry a heavy pack throughout the hike, wear the pack during long walks for a couple of

workout q&a

 Q: I've read that I should eat more salt if I'll be hiking in the heat for a few hours. Won't that extra sodium give me high blood pressure?

 A: Probably not. Case studies done at the Gatorade Sports Science Institute in Barrington, Illinois, have found that on average, people sweat anywhere from 800 to 1,400 milligrams of sodium per liter of sweat. And during a long hike, you may lose well over the recommended sodium intake of less than 2,400 milligrams a day. Most people consume 3,000 to more than 5,000 milligrams of sodium daily.

If you follow an otherwise healthful diet full of fruits, vegetables, and whole grains, a little extra salt (sodium) during your hike probably won't hurt you. On the other hand, if your doctor has restricted your salt intake because you already have high blood pressure, heed your doctor's advice.

weeks before you actually hit the trail. This will get your neck, back, and shoulders in shape.

Learn to secure your food. If you plan to camp in the wilderness, bring a nylon bag and rope to hang your food from tree branches. While it may seem logical to stash food in your tent, think about what kinds of animals wander about. You don't want a bear sniffing around your tent in the middle of the night. Stash the clothes you wore while cooking in the nylon bag as well. Otherwise, you'll smell like food and attract a sniffing animal.

Index

Underscored references indicate boxed text. **Boldface** references indicate illustrations.